Healthy and Vegetarian Cooking

100 quick and easy recipes

Maddy Curtis

Introduction

In the culinary world, there's a common notion suggesting a gap between what's healthy and what's tasty. However, plant-based cuisine challenges this assumption, demonstrating that health and pleasure can coexist harmoniously on our plates. With a wide array of fresh vegetables, legumes, whole grains, and aromatic spices, plant-based cuisine offers endless possibilities to create delicious and nutritious dishes.

Initially, there might be some skepticism towards embracing a more vegetable-based diet. However, once you delve into the world of flavors and textures offered by vegetables, you quickly discover that this cuisine is anything but bland or tasteless. On the contrary, the art of combining fresh and colorful ingredients, enhanced by creative aromas and seasonings, transforms eating into a gratifying sensory experience.

Beyond the pleasure of the palate, plant-based cuisine brings with it a host of health benefits that cannot be overlooked. Vegetables are rich in vitamins, minerals, antioxidants, and fiber, promoting the health of both body and mind. From improving digestion to reducing the risk of chronic diseases, adopting a diet rich in vegetables can lead to a healthier and more vibrant life.

In this book, we will explore the fascinating and delightful world of healthy and vegetable-based cooking. Each recipe will be a celebration of the beauty and goodness of vegetables, demonstrating that nourishing the body with natural and nutritious ingredients can be a rewarding and fulfilling experience. Whether you're a culinary expert or a beginner in search of inspiration, I invite you to join us on this culinary journey and discover the pleasure of a cuisine that nourishes not only the body but also the soul. Bon appétit!

Index

Chapter 1: *Breakfast Delights*

1. Avocado toast with cherry tomatoes 11
2. Vegan Blueberry Pancakes 12
3. Quinoa Breakfast Bowl 13
4. Green Smoothie Bowl 14
5. Tofu Scramble with Spinach 15
6. Chia Seed Pudding with Fresh Fruit 16
7. Vegan Banana Bread 17
8. Sweet Potato Hash 18
9. Breakfast Burrito with Black Beans 19
10. Overnight Oats with Almond Milk 20

Chapter 2: *Appetizers and Snacks*

11. Guacamole with Homemade Tortilla Chips 22
12. Roasted Chickpeas with Mediterranean Spices 23
13. Stuffed Mushrooms with Quinoa and Spinach 24
14. Cucumber and Hummus Roll-Ups 25
15. Caprese Skewers with Balsamic Glaze 26
16. Vegan Spinach Artichoke Dip 27
17. Edamame Salad with Ginger-Soy Dressing 28
18. Sweet Potato Fries with Garlic Aioli 29
19. Vegan Spring Rolls with Peanut Sauce 30
20. Bruschetta with Tomato and Basil 31

Chapter 3: *Soups and Salads*

21. Lentil Soup with Vegetables 33
22. Kale Caesar Salad with Avocado Dressing 34
23. Minestrone Soup with Whole Wheat Pasta 35
24. Quinoa Salad with Roasted Vegetables 36
25. Gazpacho with Fresh Herbs 37
26. Thai Coconut Curry Soup 38
27. Mediterranean Chickpea Salad 39
28. Roasted Beet Salad with Goat Cheese 40
29. Butternut Squash Soup with Sage 41
30. Greek Salad with Tofu Feta 42

Chapter 4: *Main Dishes - Pasta and Grains*

31. Spaghetti Aglio e Olio with Cherry Tomatoes 44
32. Vegan Pad Thai with Tofu 45
33. Mushroom Risotto with Arborio Rice 46

34. Quinoa Stuffed Peppers 47

35. Veggie Stir-Fry with Brown Rice 48

36. Spinach and Ricotta Stuffed Shells 49

37. Eggplant Parmesan with Marinara Sauce.. 50

38. Lemon Garlic Orzo with Asparagus... 51

39. Vegan Chili with Kidney Beans.. 52

40. Zucchini Noodles with Pesto 53

Chapter 5: *Main Dishes - Protein Alternatives*

41. Black Bean and Sweet Potato Tacos... 55

42. Lentil Shepherd's Pie... 55

43. Tempeh Stir-Fry with Ginger-Sesame Sauce 57

44. BBQ Jackfruit Sandwiches 58

45. Chickpea Tikka Masala... 59

46. Tofu and Vegetable Stir-Fry with Peanut Sauce 60

47. Quinoa and Black Bean Enchiladas 61

48. Portobello Mushroom Burgers with Avocado 62

49. Vegan Sloppy Joes with Lentils... 63

50. Cauliflower Steak with Chimichurri Sauce.. 64

Chapter 6: *Sides and Accompaniments*

51. Garlic Roasted Brussels Sprouts 66

52. Quinoa Pilaf with Herbs.. 67

53. Balsamic Glazed Carrots.. 68

54. Grilled Asparagus with Lemon Zest 69

55. Mashed Cauliflower with Vegan Butter... 70

56. Roasted Sweet Potatoes with Rosemary 71

57. Sauteed Green Beans with Almonds... 72

58. Lemon Herb Couscous... 73

59. Stuffed Bell Peppers with Quinoa and Vegetables 74

60. Vegan Cornbread with Maple Butter.. 75

Chapter 7: *Light Meals and Bowls*

61. Buddha Bowl with Quinoa, Avocado, and Chickpeas...................................... 77

62. Veggie Sushi Bowl with Brown Rice 78

63. Mediterranean Farro Salad... 79

64. Sweet Potato and Black Bean Buddha Bowl 80

65. Greek Couscous Salad with Tofu Feta.. 81

66. Southwest Quinoa Salad with Avocado Dressing.. 82

67. Asian Noodle Bowl with Tofu and Veggies 83

68. Rainbow Veggie Bowl with Turmeric Tahini Dressing.................................... 84

69. Caprese Quinoa Bowl with Balsamic Glaze 85

70. Falafel Bowl with Hummus and Tahini Sauce.. 86

Chapter 8: **Baked Goods and Desserts**

71. Vegan Chocolate Chip Cookies 88
72. Banana Bread Muffins with Walnuts 89
73. Apple Cinnamon Oatmeal Cookies 90
74. Carrot Cake Cupcakes with Cashew Cream Frosting 91
75. Blueberry Almond Flour Muffins 92
76. Vegan Chocolate Avocado Pudding 93
77. Pumpkin Spice Energy Balls 94
78. Raspberry Lemon Scones 95
79. Coconut Flour Banana Bread 96
80. Almond Butter Chocolate Chip Blondies 97

Chapter 9: **Beverages and Smoothies**

81. Green Detox Smoothie 99
82. Golden Milk Latte with Turmeric 100
83. Berry Blast Smoothie with Spinach 101
84. Iced Matcha Latte 102
85. Pineapple Mango Smoothie with Coconut Milk 103
86. Beetroot and Berry Smoothie 104
87. Cucumber Mint Lemonade 105
88. Vegan Pumpkin Spice Latte 106
89. Watermelon Cucumber Cooler 107
90. Kiwi Kale Smoothie with Ginger 108

Chapter 10: **Sauces, Dressings, and Condiments**

91. Classic Marinara Sauce 110
92. Vegan Cashew Cheese Sauce 111
93. Homemade Pesto with Basil and Pine Nuts 112
94. Balsamic Vinaigrette Dressing 113
95. Tahini Garlic Sauce 114
96 Vegan Ranch Dressing 115
97. Chimichurri Sauce with Fresh Herbs 116
98. Maple Dijon Dressing 117
99. Sriracha Mayo 118
100. Avocado Lime Crema 119

RECIPES

Chapter 1

Breakfast Delights

1. Avocado toast with cherry tomatoes

- Preparation time: 5 minutes
- Cooking time: N/A
- Portions: 2 servings

Ingredients and quantity:
- 2 slices of whole grain bread
- 1 ripe avocado
- 1 cup cherry tomatoes, halved
- Olive oil
- Salt and pepper to taste

Procedure:
1. Toast the slices of whole grain bread until golden brown.
2. Mash the ripe avocado and spread it evenly onto the toasted bread slices.
3. Top the avocado toast with halved cherry tomatoes.
4. Drizzle with olive oil and season with salt and pepper to taste.

Nutritional values:
- Calories: 200 per serving
- Protein: 6g
- Fat: 10g
- Carbohydrates: 25g
- Fiber: 8g

Shopping list:
- Whole grain bread
- Ripe avocado
- Cherry tomatoes
- Olive oil
- Salt
- Pepper

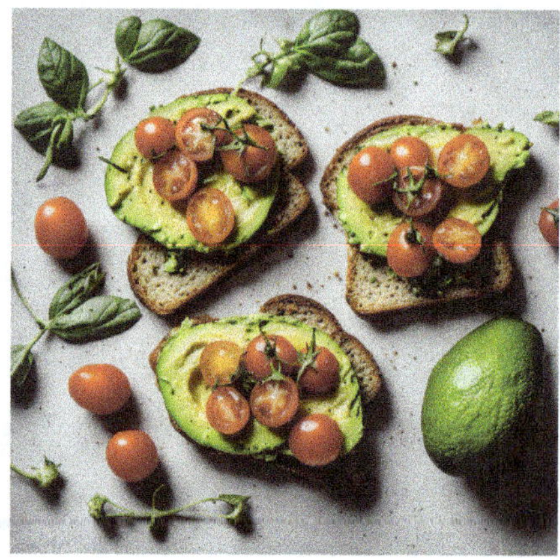

2. Vegan Blueberry Pancakes

- Preparation time: 10 minutes
- Cooking time: 15 minutes
- Portions: 4 servings

Ingredients and quantity:
- 1 1/2 cups all-purpose flour
- 2 tablespoons sugar
- 2 teaspoons baking powder
- 1/2 teaspoon salt
- 1 1/4 cups plant-based milk
  (such as almond or soy milk)
- 2 tablespoons vegetable oil
- 1 cup fresh blueberries

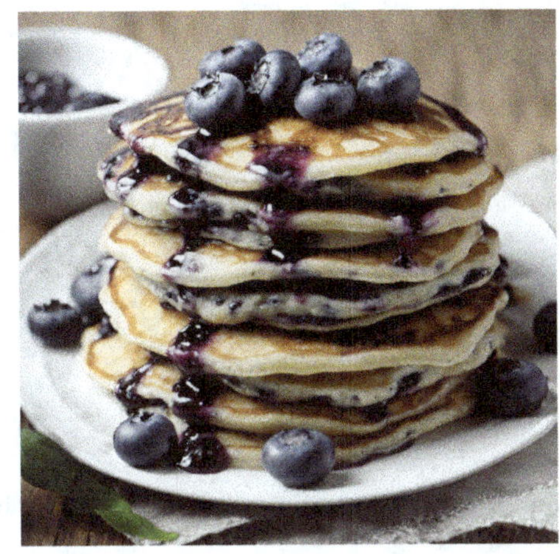

Procedure:
1. In a large bowl, whisk together the flour, sugar, baking powder, and salt.
2. In another bowl, mix the plant-based milk and vegetable oil.
3. Pour the wet ingredients into the dry ingredients and stir until just combined.
4. Gently fold in the blueberries.
5. Heat a non-stick skillet over medium heat and lightly grease with oil.
6. Pour 1/4 cup of batter onto the skillet for each pancake.
7. Cook until bubbles form on the surface, then flip and cook until golden brown.

Nutritional values:
- Calories: 220 per serving
- Protein: 5g
- Fat: 6g
- Carbohydrates: 35g
- Fiber: 2g

Shopping list:
- All-purpose flour
- Sugar
- Baking powder
- Salt
- Plant-based milk
- Vegetable oil
- Fresh blueberries

3. Quinoa Breakfast Bowl

- Preparation time: 5 minutes
- Cooking time: 15 minutes
- Portions: 2 servings

Ingredients and quantity:
 - 1 cup quinoa, rinsed
 - 2 cups water or vegetable broth
 - 1 ripe banana, sliced
 - 1/4 cup chopped almonds
 - 1 tablespoon honey or maple syrup

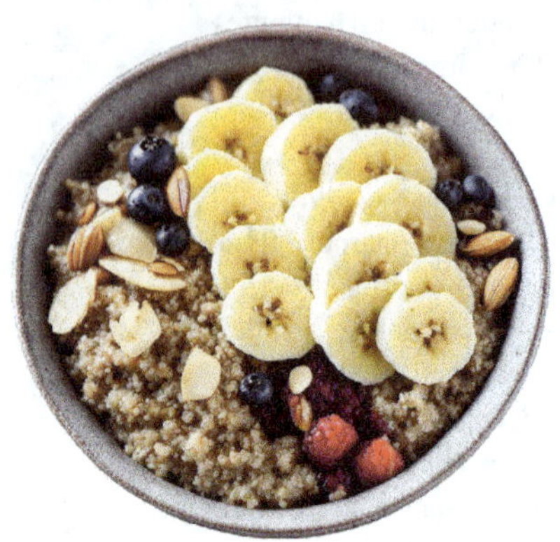

Procedure

1. In a medium saucepan, bring the water or vegetable broth to a boil.
2. Add the quinoa, reduce heat to low, and simmer covered for 15 minutes or until quinoa   is cooked and water is absorbed.
3. Divide the cooked quinoa into bowls.
4. Top with sliced banana, chopped almonds, and a drizzle of honey or maple syrup.

Nutritional values:
 - Calories: 350 per serving
 - Protein: 10g
 - Fat: 8g
 - Carbohydrates: 60g
 - Fiber: 6g

Shopping list:
 - Quinoa
 - Banana
 - Almonds
 - Honey or maple syrup

4. Green Smoothie Bowl

- Preparation time: 5 minutes
- Cooking time: N/A
- Portions: 1 serving

Ingredients and quantity:
- 1 ripe banana
- 1 cup fresh spinach leaves
- 1/2 cup chopped pineapple
- 1/2 cup coconut water or plant-based milk
- Toppings: granola, sliced kiwi, shredded coconut, chia seeds

Procedure:
1. In a blender, combine the banana, spinach, pineapple, and coconut water or plant-based milk.
2. Blend until smooth.
3. Pour the smoothie into a bowl.
4. Top with granola, sliced kiwi, shredded coconut, and chia seeds.

Nutritional values:
- Calories: 300 per serving
- Protein: 5g
- Fat: 3g
- Carbohydrates: 65g
- Fiber: 10g

Shopping list:
- Banana
- Fresh spinach leaves
- Pineapple

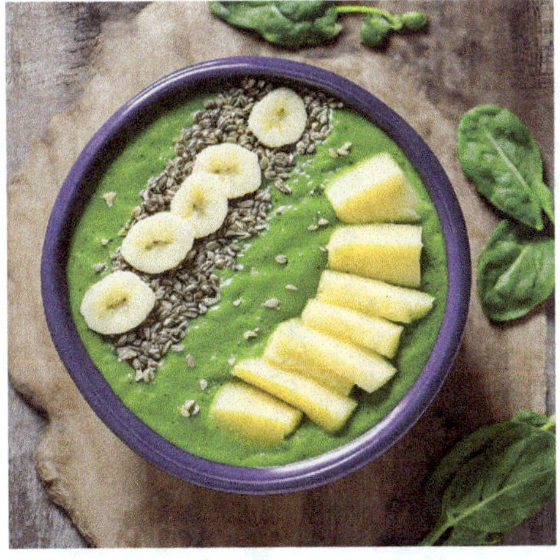

5. Tofu Scramble with Spinach

- Preparation time: 10 minutes
- Cooking time: 10 minutes
- Portions: 2 servings

Ingredients and quantity:
- 1 block (14 oz) firm tofu, drained
  and crumbled
- 2 cups fresh spinach leaves
- 1 small onion, diced
- 2 cloves garlic, minced
- 1/2 teaspoon ground turmeric
- Salt and pepper to taste
- Olive oil for cooking

Procedure:
1. Heat olive oil in a skillet over medium heat.
2. Add the diced onion and minced garlic, and
   sauté until softened.
3. Add the crumbled tofu to the skillet and
   sprinkle with ground turmeric.
4. Cook, stirring occasionally, until tofu is
   heated through and slightly browned.
5. Add the fresh spinach leaves and cook until
   wilted.
6. Season with salt and pepper to taste.

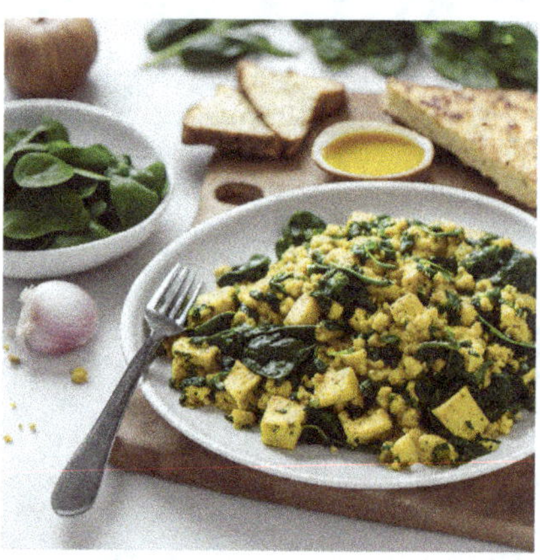

Nutritional values:
- Calories: 200 per serving
- Protein: 15g
- Fat: 10g
- Carbohydrates: 10g
- Fiber: 4g

Shopping list:
- Firm tofu
- Fresh spinach leaves
- Onion
- Garlic
- Ground turmeric
- Olive oil

6. Chia Seed Pudding with Fresh Fruit

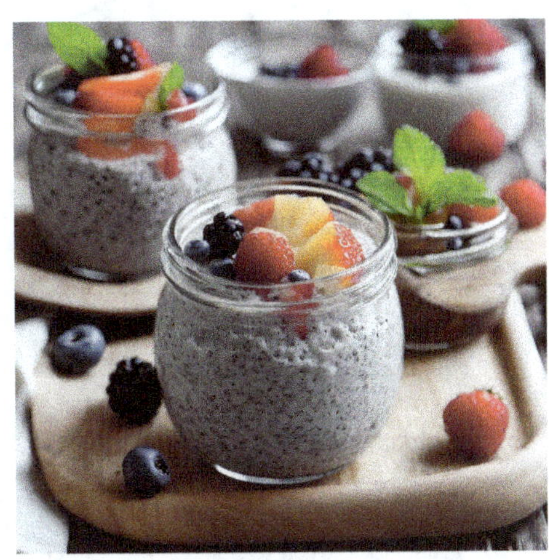

- Preparation time: 5 minutes
  - Cooking time: 0 minutes
    (overnight chilling)
  - Portions: 2 servings

Ingredients and quantity:
  - 1/4 cup chia seeds
  - 1 cup almond milk or any plant-based milk
  - 1 tablespoon maple syrup or honey
  - 1/2 teaspoon vanilla extract
  - Fresh fruit for topping
    (e.g., berries, sliced banana)

Procedure:
1. In a bowl, mix together chia seeds, almond milk, maple syrup or honey, and vanilla extract.
2. Cover and refrigerate overnight or for at least 4 hours, until thickened.
3. Divide the pudding into serving bowls and top with fresh fruit before serving.

Nutritional values:
  - Calories: 150 per serving
  - Protein: 5g
  - Fat: 7g
  - Carbohydrates: 20g
  - Fiber: 10g

Shopping list:
  - Chia seeds
  - Almond milk or any plant-based milk
  - Maple syrup or honey
  - Vanilla extract
  - Fresh fruit (e.g., berries, banana)

7. Vegan Banana Bread

- Preparation time: 15 minutes
- Cooking time: 1 hour
- Portions: 8 servings

Ingredients and quantity:
  - 3 ripe bananas, mashed
  - 1/4 cup coconut oil, melted
  - 1/2 cup coconut sugar or brown sugar
  - 1 teaspoon vanilla extract
  - 1 1/2 cups all-purpose flour
  - 1 teaspoon baking soda
  - 1/2 teaspoon salt

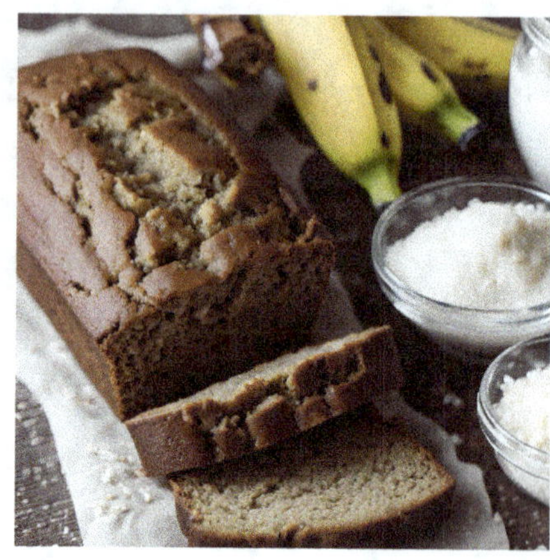

Procedure:
  1. Preheat the oven to 350°F (175°C). Grease a
     loaf pan with coconut oil or line with parchment paper.
  2. In a large mixing bowl, combine mashed bananas, melted coconut oil, coconut sugar or
     brown sugar, and vanilla extract.
  3. In a separate bowl, whisk together the flour, baking soda, and salt.
  4. Gradually add the dry ingredients to the wet ingredients, stirring until just combined.
  5. Pour the batter into the prepared loaf pan and spread it evenly.
  6. Bake for 50-60 minutes, or until a toothpick inserted into the center comes out clean.
  7. Allow the banana bread to cool in the pan for 10 minutes before transferring it to a wire rack to
     cool completely.

Nutritional values:
  - Calories: 250 per serving
  - Protein: 3g
  - Fat: 10g
  - Carbohydrates: 40g
  - Fiber: 3g

Shopping list:
  - Ripe bananas
  - Coconut oil
  - Coconut sugar or brown sugar
  - Vanilla extract
  - All-purpose flour
  - Baking soda
  - Salt

8. Sweet Potato Hash

- Preparation time: 10 minutes
- Cooking time: 20 minutes
- Portions: 4 servings

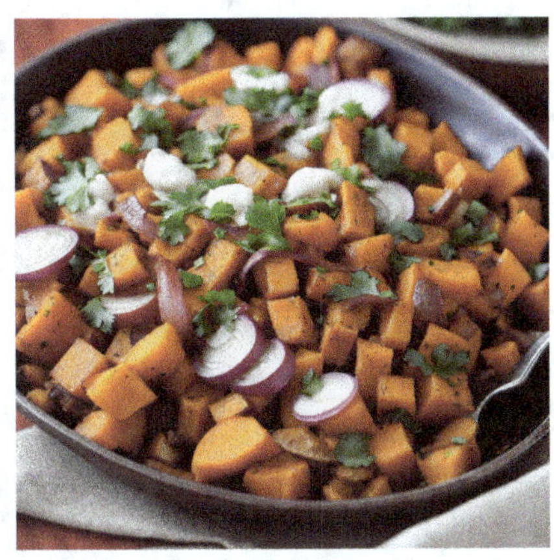

Ingredients and quantity:
- 2 medium sweet potatoes, peeled and diced
- 1 small onion, diced
- 1 bell pepper, diced
- 2 cloves garlic, minced
- 1 teaspoon smoked paprika
- Salt and pepper to taste
- Olive oil for cooking

Procedure:
1. Heat olive oil in a skillet over medium heat.
2. Add the diced sweet potatoes and cook until tender and lightly browned, about 10 minutes.
3. Add the diced onion, bell pepper, and minced garlic to the skillet. Cook until the vegetables are softened.
4. Sprinkle with smoked paprika, salt, and pepper, and cook for an additional 2-3 minutes.

Nutritional values:
- Calories: 180 per serving
- Protein: 3g
- Fat: 5g
- Carbohydrates: 30g
- Fiber: 5g

Shopping list:
- Sweet potatoes
- Onion
- Bell pepper
- Garlic
- Smoked paprika
- Olive oil

9. Breakfast Burrito with Black Beans

- Preparation time: 10 minutes
- Cooking time: 10 minutes
- Portions: 2 servings

Ingredients and quantity:
- 4 large flour tortillas
- 1 cup cooked black beans
- 4 large eggs, beaten
- 1/2 cup shredded vegan cheese
- 1 avocado, sliced
- Salsa, for serving

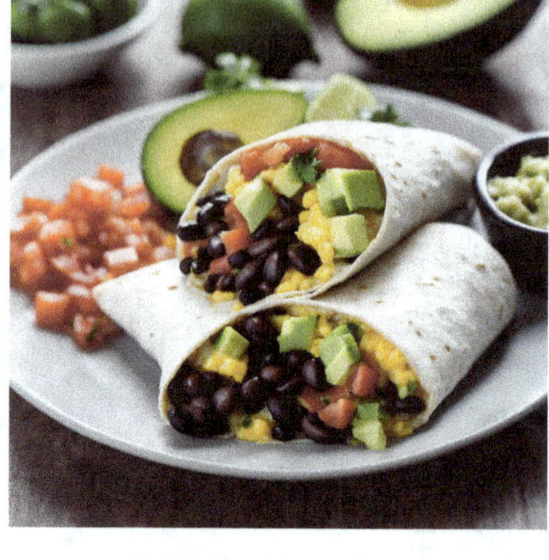

Procedure:
1. Heat the tortillas in a skillet or microwave until warm and pliable.
2. In a separate skillet, scramble the eggs until cooked through.
3. Assemble the burritos by layering the cooked black beans, scrambled eggs, vegan cheese, and sliced avocado on each tortilla.
4. Roll up the tortillas tightly to form burritos.
5. Serve with salsa on the side.

Nutritional values:
- Calories: 400 per serving
- Protein: 20g
- Fat: 15g
- Carbohydrates: 45g
- Fiber: 10g

Shopping list:
- Flour tortillas
- Cooked black beans
- Eggs
- Vegan cheese
- Avocado
- Salsa

10. Overnight Oats with Almond Milk

- Preparation time: 5 minutes
  - Cooking time: N/A (overnight soaking)
  - Portions: 2 servings

Ingredients and quantity:
  - 1 cup rolled oats
  - 1 cup almond milk (or any plant-based milk)
  - 2 tablespoons chia seeds
  - 1 tablespoon maple syrup or honey
  - 1/2 teaspoon vanilla extract
  - Toppings: sliced bananas, berries, nuts, seeds

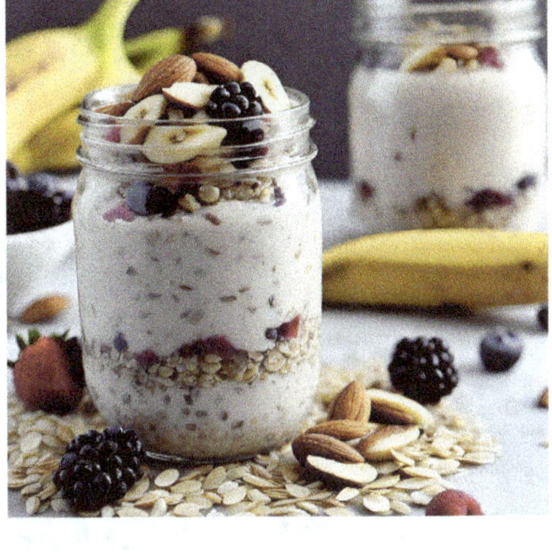

Procedure:
  1. In a jar or bowl, combine the rolled oats, almond
     milk, chia seeds, maple syrup
     or honey, and vanilla extract.
  2. Stir well to combine all ingredients.
  3. Cover and refrigerate overnight, or for at least 4 hours.
  4. Before serving, give the overnight oats a good stir and add your favorite toppings,
     such as sliced bananas, berries, nuts, or seeds.

Nutritional values:
  - Calories: 250 per serving
  - Protein: 8g
  - Fat: 6g
  - Carbohydrates: 40g
  - Fiber: 8g

Shopping list:
  - Rolled oats
  - Almond milk or any plant-based milk
  - Chia seeds
  - Maple syrup or honey
  - Vanilla extract
  - Sliced bananas
  - Berries
  - Nuts
  - Seeds

Appetizers and Snacks

11. Guacamole with Homemade Tortilla Chips

- Preparation time: 15 minutes
- Cooking time: 10 minutes
- Portions: 4 servings

Ingredients and quantity:
  - 3 ripe avocados
  - 1 tomato, diced
  - 1/4 cup red onion, finely chopped
  - 1/4 cup fresh cilantro, chopped
  - 1 lime, juiced
  - Salt and pepper to taste
  - 4 corn tortillas
  - Olive oil spray

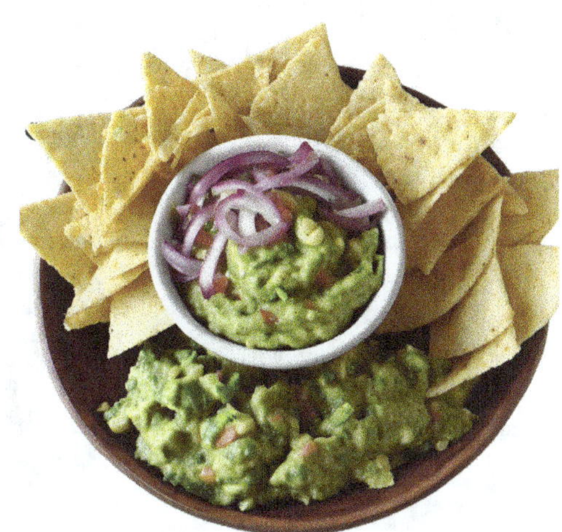

Procedure:
1. In a bowl, mash the avocados with a fork until smooth.
2. Add the diced tomato, chopped red onion, chopped cilantro, lime juice, salt, and pepper to the mashed avocados. Mix until well combined.
3. Preheat the oven to 375°F (190°C).
4. Cut the corn tortillas into triangles and place them on a baking sheet lined with parchment paper.
5. Lightly spray the tortilla triangles with olive oil and sprinkle with salt.
6. Bake in the preheated oven for 8-10 minutes, or until crispy and golden brown.
7. Serve the guacamole with the homemade tortilla chips.

Nutritional values:
  - Guacamole (per serving):
  - Calories: 180
  - Protein: 3g
  - Fat: 15g
  - Carbohydrates: 12g
  - Fiber: 8g
  - Tortilla chips (per serving):
  - Calories: 80
  - Protein: 2g
  - Fat: 2g
  - Carbohydrates: 15g
  - Fiber: 2g

Shopping list:
  - Ripe avocados
  - Tomato
  - Red onion
  - Fresh cilantro
  - Lime
  - Corn tortillas
  - Olive oil spray

12. Roasted Chickpeas with Mediterranean Spices

- Preparation time: 5 minutes
- Cooking time: 30 minutes (may vary depending on oven and desired crispiness)
- Portions: 4 servings

Ingredients and quantity:
- 2 cans (15 oz each) chickpeas, drained and rinsed
- 2 tablespoons olive oil
- 1 teaspoon ground cumin
- 1 teaspoon paprika
- 1/2 teaspoon garlic powder
- 1/2 teaspoon onion powder
- Salt and pepper to taste

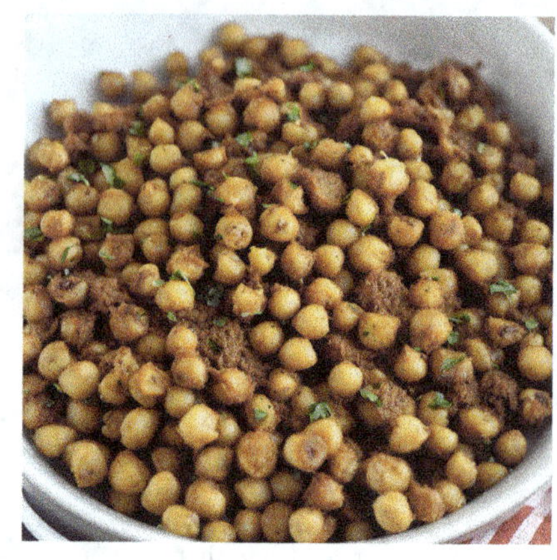

Procedure:
1. Preheat the oven to 400°F (200°C). Line a baking sheet with parchment paper.
2. In a large bowl, toss the drained and rinsed chickpeas with olive oil until evenly coated.
3. Add the ground cumin, paprika, garlic powder, onion powder, salt, and pepper. Toss until the chickpeas are evenly seasoned.
4. Spread the seasoned chickpeas in a single layer on the prepared baking sheet.
5. Roast in the preheated oven for 25-30 minutes, shaking the pan halfway through, until the chickpeas are crispy and golden brown.
6. Remove from the oven and let cool slightly before serving.

Nutritional values (per serving):
- Calories: 210
- Protein: 9g
- Fat: 8g
- Carbohydrates: 28g
- Fiber: 8g

Shopping list:
- Canned chickpeas
- Olive oil
- Ground cumin
- Paprika
- Garlic powder
- Onion powder
- Salt
- Pepper

13. Stuffed Mushrooms with Quinoa and Spinach

- Preparation time: 15 minutes
- Cooking time: 20 minutes
- Portions: 4 servings

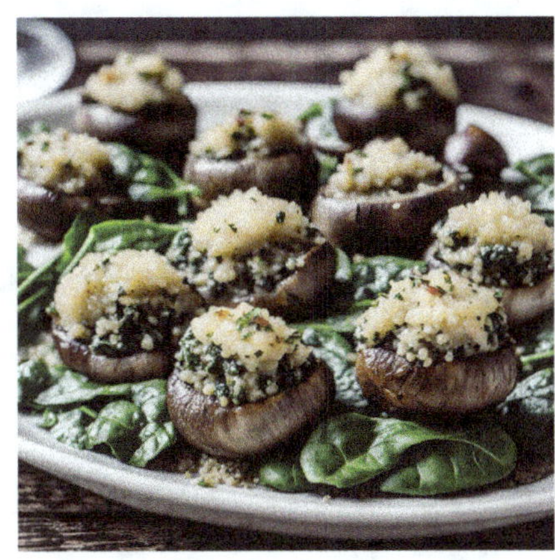

Ingredients and quantity:
- 12 large mushrooms, stems removed and finely chopped
- 1 cup cooked quinoa
- 1 cup fresh spinach, chopped
- 1/4 cup red onion, finely chopped
- 2 cloves garlic, minced
- 1/4 cup vegan parmesan cheese, grated
- Salt and pepper to taste
- Olive oil for cooking

Procedure:
1. Preheat the oven to 375°F (190°C). Line a baking sheet with parchment paper.
2. In a skillet, heat olive oil over medium heat. Add the chopped mushroom stems, red onion, and garlic. Cook until softened.
3. Add the cooked quinoa and chopped spinach to the skillet. Cook until the spinach wilts.
4. Remove the skillet from heat and stir in the vegan parmesan cheese. Season with salt and pepper to taste.
5. Stuff each mushroom cap with the quinoa and spinach mixture.
6. Place the stuffed mushrooms on the prepared baking sheet and bake for 15-20 minutes, or until mushrooms are tender.

Nutritional values (per serving):
- Calories: 150
- Protein: 6g
- Fat: 4g
- Carbohydrates: 23g
- Fiber: 5g

Shopping list:
- Large mushrooms
- Cooked quinoa
- Fresh spinach
- Red onion
- Garlic
- Vegan parmesan cheese
- Olive oil

14. Cucumber and Hummus Roll-Ups

- Preparation time: 10 minutes
  - Cooking time: 0 minutes
  - Portions: 4 servings

Ingredients and quantity:
  - 2 large cucumbers
  - 1/2 cup hummus
  - 1/4 cup roasted red peppers, sliced
  - 1/4 cup baby spinach leaves
  - Salt and pepper to taste

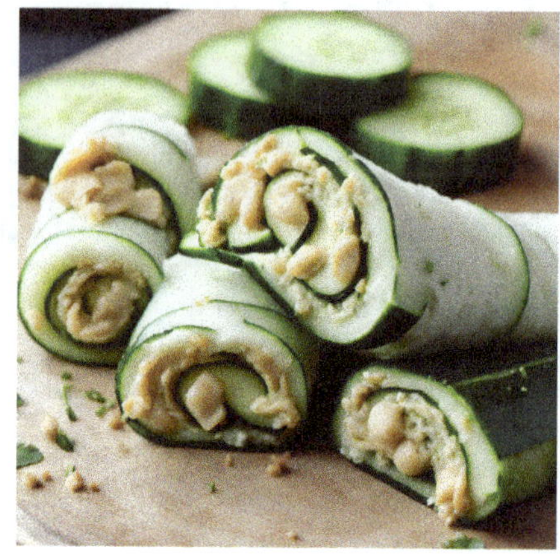

Procedure:
  1. Use a vegetable peeler to slice the cucumbers lengthwise into thin strips.
  2. Spread a thin layer of hummus onto each cucumber strip.
  3. Place a few slices of roasted red peppers and a couple of spinach leaves at one end of each cucumber strip.
  4. Roll up the cucumber strips tightly to form roll-ups.
  5. Secure the roll-ups with toothpicks if needed.
  6. Season with salt and pepper to taste.

Nutritional values (per serving):
  - Calories: 70
  - Protein: 3g
  - Fat: 3g
  - Carbohydrates: 9g
  - Fiber: 3g

Shopping list:
- Large cucumbers
- Hummus
- Roasted

15. Caprese Skewers with Balsamic Glaze

- Preparation time: 15 minutes
- Cooking time: 0 minutes
- Portions: 4 servings

Ingredients and quantity:
  - 1 pint cherry tomatoes
  - 8 oz fresh mozzarella cheese,
    cut into bite-sized pieces
  - Fresh basil leaves
  - Balsamic glaze
  - Salt and pepper to taste
  - Toothpicks or skewers

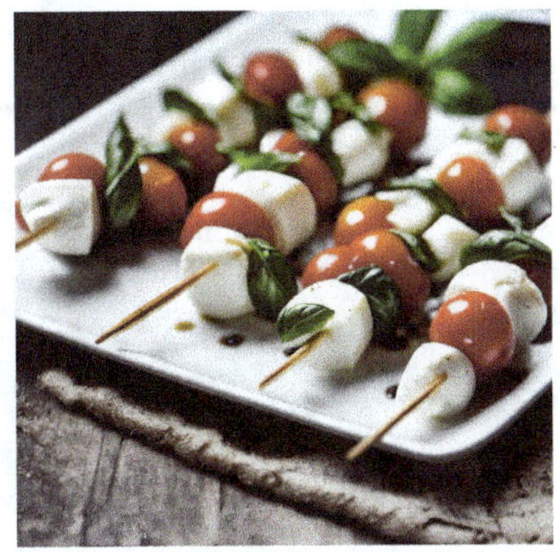

Procedure:
  1. Thread one cherry tomato, one piece of mozzarella cheese, and one basil leaf onto
     each toothpick or skewer.
  2. Repeat until all ingredients are used.
  3. Arrange the skewers on a serving platter.
  4. Drizzle with balsamic glaze.
  5. Season with salt and pepper to taste.

Nutritional values (per serving):
  - Calories: 120
  - Protein: 8g
  - Fat: 7g
  - Carbohydrates: 7g
  - Fiber: 1g

Shopping list:
  - Cherry tomatoes
  - Fresh mozzarella cheese
  - Fresh basil leaves
  - Balsamic glaze
  - Toothpicks or skewers

16. Vegan Spinach Artichoke Dip

- Preparation time: 10 minutes
- Cooking time: 20 minutes
- Portions: 6 servings

Ingredients and quantity:
  - 1 cup raw cashews, soaked overnight
    and drained
  - 1 tablespoon olive oil
  - 1 small onion, diced
  - 2 cloves garlic, minced
  - 1 can (14 oz) artichoke hearts,
    drained and chopped
  - 2 cups fresh spinach, chopped
  - 1/4 cup nutritional yeast
  - 1/2 cup vegetable broth
  - Salt and pepper to taste

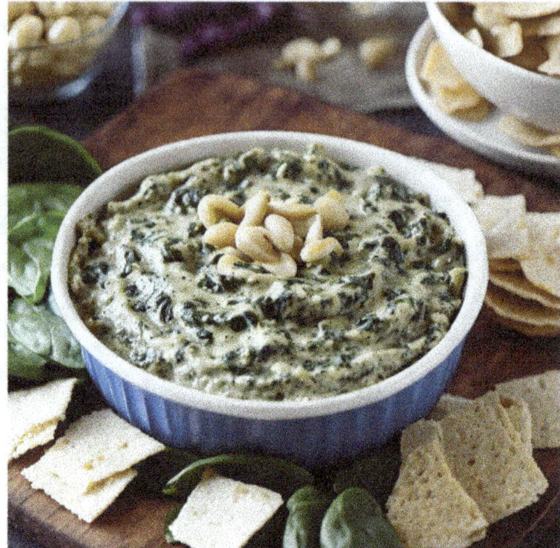

Procedure:
  1. Preheat the oven to 375°F (190°C).
  2. In a skillet, heat olive oil over medium heat. Add the diced onion and minced garlic.
     Cook until softened.
  3. Add the chopped artichoke hearts and chopped spinach to the skillet. Cook until
     the spinach wilts.
  4. In a blender, combine the soaked cashews, cooked vegetable mixture, nutritional yeast,
     and vegetable broth. Blend until smooth and creamy.
  5. Transfer the mixture to an oven-safe baking dish.
  6. Bake in the preheated oven for 20 minutes, or until bubbly and lightly golden on top.

Nutritional values (per serving):
  - Calories: 180
  - Protein: 7g
  - Fat: 12g
  - Carbohydrates: 14g
  - Fiber: 4g

Shopping list:
  - Raw cashews
  - Olive oil
  - Onion
  - Garlic
  - Canned artichoke hearts
  - Fresh spinach
  - Nutritional yeast
  - Vegetable broth

17. Edamame Salad with Ginger-Soy Dressing

- Preparation time: 10 minutes
- Cooking time: 5 minutes
- Portions: 4 servings

Ingredients and quantity:
  - 2 cups shelled edamame, cooked
  - 1 red bell pepper, diced
  - 1 cup shredded carrots
  - 1/4 cup chopped cilantro
  - 2 tablespoons sesame oil
  - 1 tablespoon soy sauce
  - 1 tablespoon rice vinegar
  - 1 teaspoon fresh ginger, grated
  - 1 teaspoon honey or maple syrup
  - Sesame seeds for garnish

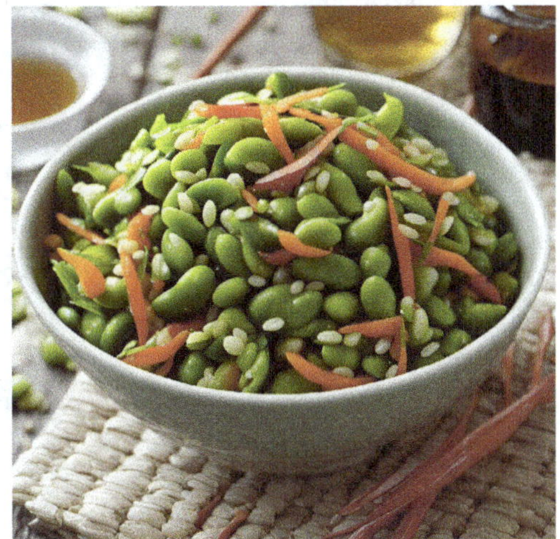

Procedure:
  1. In a large bowl, combine the cooked
     edamame, diced red bell pepper,
     shredded carrots, and chopped cilantro.
  2. In a small bowl, whisk together the sesame oil, soy sauce, rice vinegar,
     grated ginger, and honey or maple syrup to make the dressing.
  3. Pour the dressing over the salad and toss to combine.
  4. Garnish with sesame seeds before serving.

Nutritional values (per serving):
  - Calories: 180
  - Protein: 10g
  - Fat: 8g
  - Carbohydrates: 20g
  - Fiber: 6g

Shopping list:
  - Shelled edamame
  - Red bell pepper
  - Carrots
  - Cilantro
  - Sesame oil
  - Soy sauce
  - Rice vinegar
  - Fresh ginger
  - Honey or maple syrup
  - Sesame seeds

18. Sweet Potato Fries with Garlic Aioli

- Preparation time: 15 minutes
- Cooking time: 25 minutes
- Portions: 4 servings

Ingredients and quantity:
  - 2 large sweet potatoes, cut into fries
  - 2 tablespoons olive oil
  - 1 teaspoon paprika
  - 1/2 teaspoon garlic powder
  - Salt and pepper to taste
  - 1/2 cup vegan mayonnaise
  - 2 cloves garlic, minced
  - 1 tablespoon lemon juice

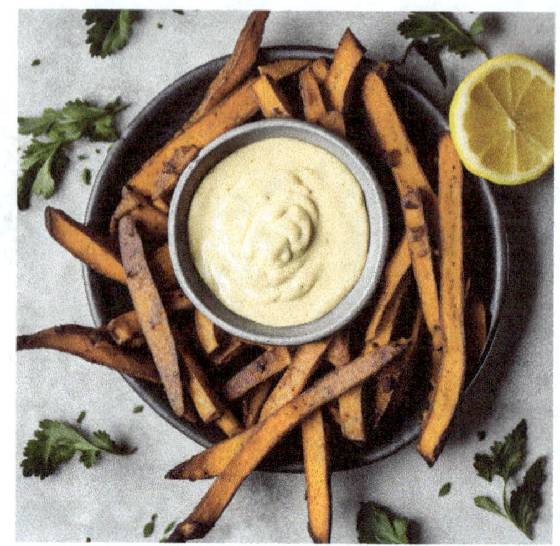

Procedure:
  1. Preheat the oven to 425°F (220°C). Line a baking sheet with parchment paper.
  2. In a large bowl, toss the sweet potato fries with olive oil, paprika, garlic powder, salt, and pepper until evenly coated.
  3. Spread the fries in a single layer on the prepared baking sheet.
  4. Bake in the preheated oven for 20-25 minutes, flipping halfway through, until the fries are golden brown and crispy.
  5. In a small bowl, whisk together the vegan mayonnaise, minced garlic, and lemon juice to make the garlic aioli.
  6. Serve the sweet potato fries with the garlic aioli on the side for dipping.

Nutritional values (per serving):
  - Calories: 220
  - Protein: 3g
  - Fat: 14g
  - Carbohydrates: 22g
  - Fiber: 4g

Shopping list:
  - Large sweet potatoes
  - Olive oil
  - Paprika
  - Garlic powder
  - Vegan mayonnaise
  - Lemon juice.

19. Vegan Spring Rolls with Peanut Sauce

- Preparation time: 20 minutes
- Cooking time: 0 minutes
- Portions: 4 servings

Ingredients and quantity:
  - 8 rice paper wrappers
  - 2 cups shredded lettuce
  - 1 cup shredded red cabbage
  - 1 carrot, julienned
  - 1 cucumber, julienned
  - 1/4 cup fresh mint leaves
  - 1/4 cup fresh cilantro leaves
  - 1/4 cup chopped peanuts
  - 1/4 cup peanut butter
  - 2 tablespoons soy sauce
  - 1 tablespoon maple syrup or honey
  - 1 tablespoon lime juice
  - 1 clove garlic, minced
  - Water for soaking rice paper wrappers

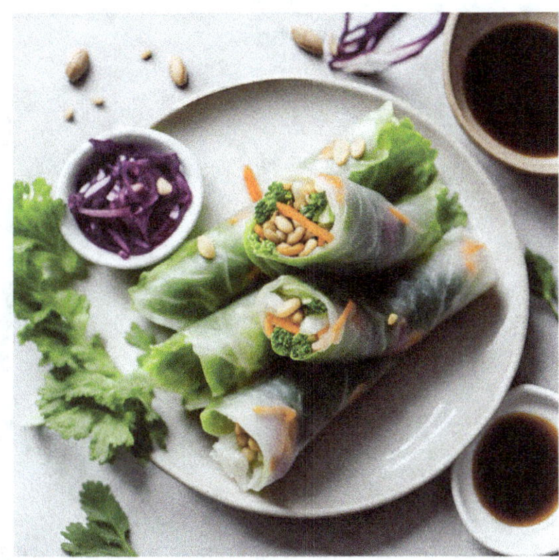

Procedure:
  1. Fill a shallow dish with warm water.
  2. Dip one rice paper wrapper into the warm water for a few seconds until softened.
  3. Place the softened rice paper wrapper on a clean surface.
  4. Layer shredded lettuce, shredded red cabbage, julienned carrot, julienned cucumber, mint leaves, cilantro leaves, and chopped peanuts on the bottom third of the rice paper wrapper.
  5. Fold the sides of the wrapper over the filling, then roll tightly to enclose the filling like a burrito.
  6. Repeat with the remaining rice paper wrappers and filling ingredients.
  7. In a small bowl, whisk together the peanut butter, soy sauce, maple syrup or honey, lime juice, and minced garlic to make the peanut sauce.
  8. Serve the spring rolls with the peanut sauce for dipping.

Nutritional values (per serving):
  - Calories: 250
  - Protein: 8g
  - Fat: 12g
  - Carbohydrates: 30g
  - Fiber: 6g

Shopping list:
  - Rice paper wrappers
  - Lettuce
  - Red cabbage
  - Carrot
  - Cucumber
  - Fresh mint leaves
  - Fresh cilantro leaves
  - Peanuts
  - Peanut butter
  - Soy sauce
  - Maple syrup or honey
  - Lime
  - Garlic.

20. Bruschetta with Tomato and Basil

- Preparation time: 10 minutes
- Cooking time: 5 minutes
- Portions: 4 servings

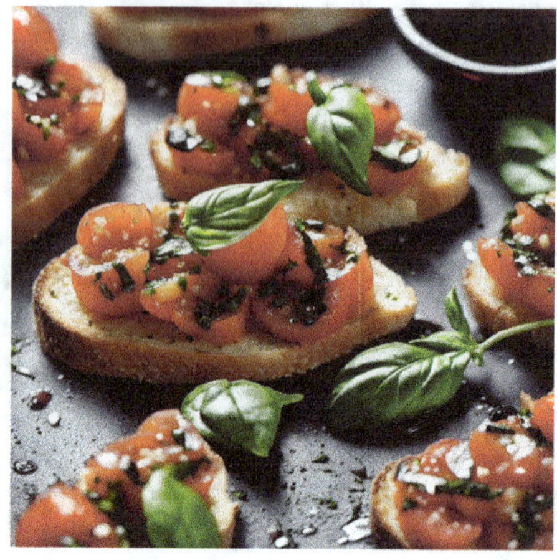

Ingredients and quantity:
  - 4 slices crusty bread, sliced diagonally
  - 2 large tomatoes, diced
  - 2 cloves garlic, minced
  - 1/4 cup fresh basil leaves, chopped
  - 2 tablespoons balsamic vinegar
  - 2 tablespoons extra virgin olive oil
  - Salt and pepper to taste

Procedure:
  1. Preheat the oven to 375°F (190°C).
  2. Place the sliced bread on a baking sheet and toast in the preheated oven for 5 minutes, or until lightly golden and crisp.
  3. In a bowl, combine the diced tomatoes, minced garlic, chopped basil leaves, balsamic vinegar, and extra virgin olive oil. Mix well.
  4. Season the tomato mixture with salt and pepper to taste.
  5. Spoon the tomato mixture evenly onto the toasted bread slices.
  6. Serve the bruschetta immediately as an appetizer or snack.

Nutritional values (per serving):
  - Calories: 180
  - Protein: 4g
  - Fat: 8g
  - Carbohydrates: 24g
  - Fiber: 3g

Shopping list:
  - Crusty bread
  - Tomatoes
  - Garlic
  - Fresh basil leaves
  - Balsamic vinegar
  - Extra virgin olive oil

Chapter 3

29

Soups and Salads

21. Lentil Soup with Vegetables

- Preparation time: 15 minutes
- Cooking time: 45 minutes
- Portions: 6 servings

Ingredients and quantity:
- 1 cup green lentils, rinsed
- 1 tablespoon olive oil
- 1 onion, diced
- 2 carrots, diced
- 2 celery stalks, diced
- 2 cloves garlic, minced
- 6 cups vegetable broth
- 1 can (14 oz) diced tomatoes
- 1 teaspoon dried thyme
- Salt and pepper to taste

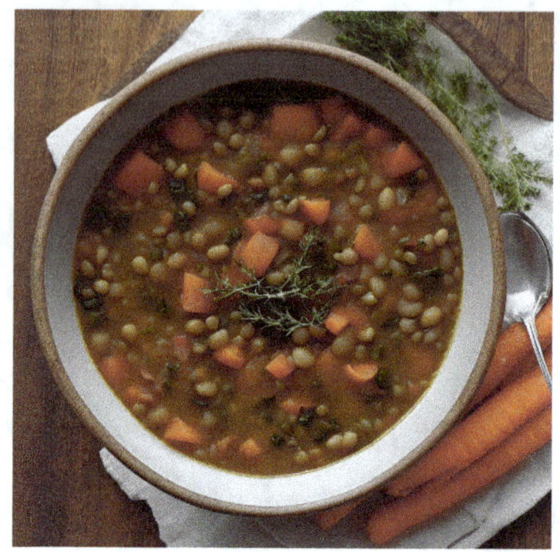

Procedure:
1. In a large pot, heat olive oil over
   medium heat. Add diced onion, carrots, celery,
   and minced garlic. Cook until softened.
2. Add rinsed lentils, vegetable broth, diced tomatoes, dried thyme, salt, and pepper
   to the pot. Bring to a boil.
3. Reduce heat to low and simmer for 30-35 minutes, or until lentils are tender.
4. Adjust seasoning if necessary and serve hot.

Nutritional values (per serving):
- Calories: 220
- Protein: 13g
- Fat: 3g
- Carbohydrates: 38g
- Fiber: 15g

Shopping list:
- Green lentils
- Olive oil
- Onion
- Carrots
- Celery
- Garlic
- Vegetable broth
- Canned diced tomatoes
- Dried thyme

22. Kale Caesar Salad with Avocado Dressing

- Preparation time: 15 minutes
- Cooking time: 0 minutes
- Portions: 4 servings

Ingredients and quantity:
- 1 bunch kale, stems removed and leaves torn into bite-sized pieces
- 1 avocado, ripe

- 2 tablespoons lemon juice
- 2 tablespoons olive oil
- 2 cloves garlic, minced
- 2 tablespoons nutritional yeast
- Salt and pepper to taste
- 1/4 cup cherry tomatoes, halved
- 1/4 cup sliced cucumber
- 1/4 cup croutons (optional)

Procedure:
1. In a large salad bowl, massage the torn kale leaves with a drizzle of olive oil for a few minutes to soften them.
2. In a blender or food processor, combine the ripe avocado, lemon juice, olive oil, minced garlic, nutritional yeast, salt, and pepper. Blend until smooth and creamy.
3. Pour the avocado dressing over the massaged kale and toss until the leaves are evenly coated.
4. Add the cherry tomatoes, sliced cucumber, and croutons (if using) to the salad and toss gently to combine.
5. Serve immediately as a light and refreshing meal.

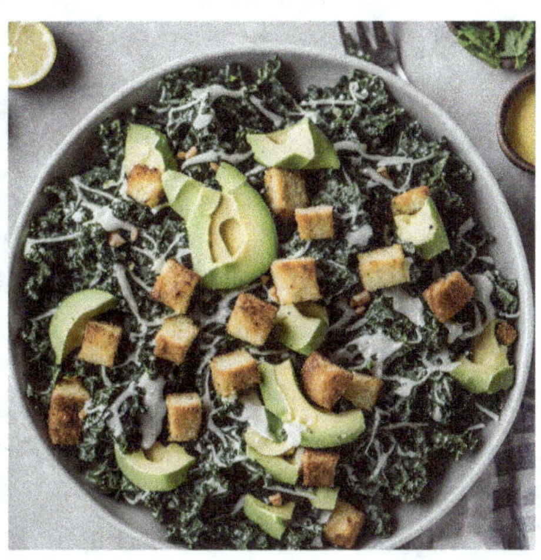

Nutritional values (per serving):
- Calories: 180
- Protein: 4g
- Fat: 13g
- Carbohydrates: 15g
- Fiber: 6g

Shopping list:
- Kale
- Avocado
- Lemon
- Olive oil
- Garlic
- Nutritional yeast
- Cherry tomatoes
- Cucumber
- Croutons (optional)

23. Minestrone Soup with Whole Wheat Pasta

- Preparation time: 15 minutes
- Cooking time: 30 minutes
- Portions: 6 servings

Ingredients and quantity:
  - 1 tablespoon olive oil
  - 1 onion, diced
  - 2 carrots, diced
  - 2 celery stalks, diced
  - 2 cloves garlic, minced
  - 6 cups vegetable broth
  - 1 can (14 oz) diced tomatoes
  - 1 can (15 oz) kidney beans,
    drained and rinsed
  - 1 cup whole wheat pasta
    (e.g., fusilli or penne)
  - 2 cups chopped spinach or kale
  - 1 teaspoon dried oregano
  - Salt and pepper to taste

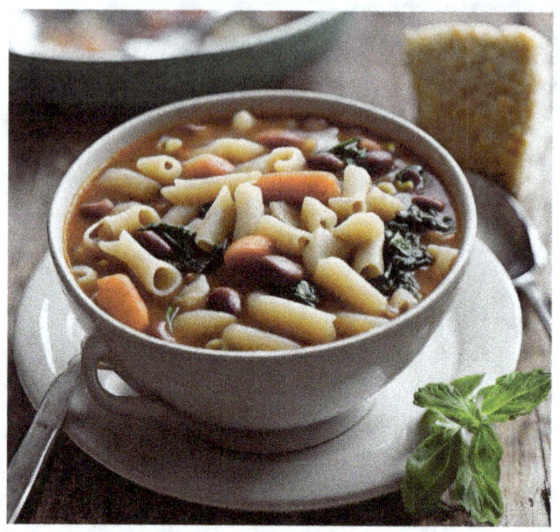

Procedure:
  1. In a large pot, heat olive oil over medium heat. Add diced onion, carrots, celery, and minced garlic. Cook until softened.
  2. Add vegetable broth, diced tomatoes, kidney beans, whole wheat pasta, dried oregano, salt, and pepper to the pot. Bring to a boil.
  3. Reduce heat to low and simmer for 15-20 minutes, or until the pasta is cooked.
  4. Stir in chopped spinach or kale and cook for an additional 5 minutes.
  5. Adjust seasoning if necessary and serve hot.

Nutritional values (per serving):
  - Calories: 280
  - Protein: 12g
  - Fat: 3g
  - Carbohydrates: 52g
  - Fiber: 10g

Shopping list:
  - Olive oil
  - Onion
  - Carrots
  - Celery
  - Garlic
  - Vegetable broth
  - Canned diced tomatoes
  - Canned kidney beans
  - Whole wheat pasta
  - Spinach or kale
  - Dried oregan

24. Quinoa Salad with Roasted Vegetables

- Preparation time: 15 minutes
- Cooking time: 25 minutes
- Portions: 4 servings

Ingredients and quantity:
- 1 cup quinoa, rinsed
- 2 cups water or vegetable broth
- 1 small sweet potato, diced
- 1 red bell pepper, diced
- 1 zucchini, diced
- 1 tablespoon olive oil
- Salt and pepper to taste
- 2 cups baby spinach
- 1/4 cup chopped fresh parsley
- 1/4 cup crumbled feta cheese (optional)
- 2 tablespoons balsamic vinegar
- 1 tablespoon Dijon mustard
- 2 tablespoons extra virgin olive oil

Procedure:
1. Preheat the oven to 400°F (200°C). Line a baking sheet with parchment paper.
2. In a medium saucepan, combine quinoa and water or vegetable broth. Bring to a boil, then reduce heat to low, cover, and simmer for 15 minutes, or until quinoa is cookedand water is absorbed.
3. Meanwhile, spread diced sweet potato, red bell pepper, and zucchini on the prepared baking sheet. Drizzle with olive oil and season with salt and pepper. Toss to coat.
4. Roast in the preheated oven for 20-25 minutes, or until vegetables are tender and lightly browned.
5. In a large salad bowl, combine cooked quinoa, roasted vegetables, baby spinach, chopped parsley, and crumbled feta cheese (if using).
6. In a small bowl, whisk together balsamic vinegar, Dijon mustard, and extra virgin olive oil to make the dressing.
7. Pour the dressing over the quinoa salad and toss to coat evenly.
8. Serve immediately or refrigerate until ready to serve.

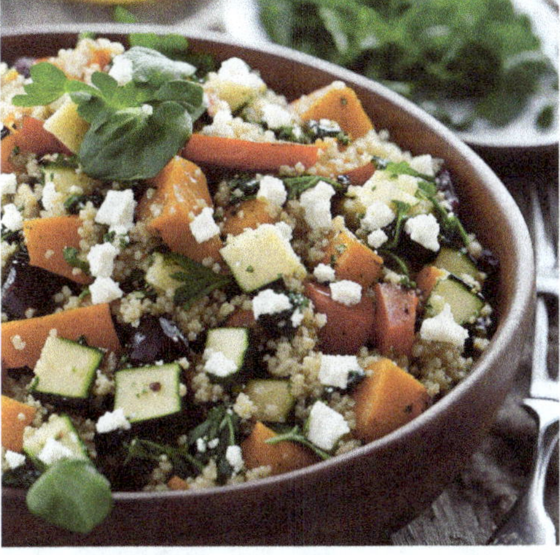

Nutritional values (per serving):
- Calories: 320
- Protein: 9g
- Fat: 14g
- Carbohydrates: 40g
- Fiber: 7g

Shopping list:
- Quinoa
- Sweet potato
- Red bell pepper
- Zucchini
- Olive oil
- Baby spinach
- Fresh parsley
- Feta cheese (optional)
- Balsamic vinegar
- Dijon mustard
- Extra virgin olive oil

25. Gazpacho with Fresh Herbs

- Preparation time: 15 minutes
- Cooking time: 0 minutes
- Portions: 4 servings

Ingredients and quantity:
- 6 ripe tomatoes, chopped
- 1 cucumber, peeled and chopped
- 1 red bell pepper, seeded and chopped
- 1 small red onion, chopped
- 2 cloves garlic, minced
- 2 tablespoons red wine vinegar
- 1/4 cup extra virgin olive oil
- 2 cups tomato juice
- 1 teaspoon salt
- 1/2 teaspoon black pepper
- 1/4 cup chopped fresh basil
- 1/4 cup chopped fresh parsley

Procedure:
1. In a blender or food processor, combine chopped tomatoes, cucumber, red bell pepper, red onion, minced garlic, red wine vinegar, and extra virgin olive oil. Blend until smooth.
2. Transfer the blended mixture to a large bowl. Stir in tomato juice, salt, and black pepper.
3. Cover and refrigerate for at least 1 hour to chill.
4. Before serving, stir in chopped fresh basil and parsley.
5. Serve the gazpacho chilled, garnished with additional herbs if desired.

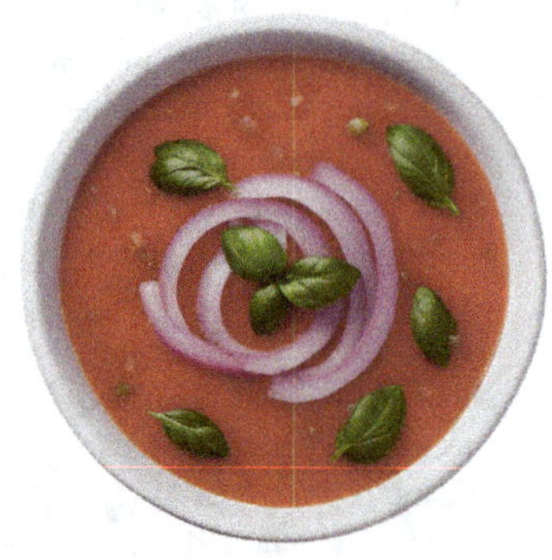

Nutritional values (per serving):
- Calories: 150
- Protein: 3g
- Fat: 10g
- Carbohydrates: 14g
- Fiber: 4g

Shopping list:
- Ripe tomatoes
- Cucumber
- Red bell pepper
- Red onion
- Garlic
- Red wine vinegar
- Extra virgin olive oil
- Tomato juice
- Fresh basil
- Fresh parsley

26. Thai Coconut Curry Soup

- Preparation time: 15 minutes
- Cooking time: 25 minutes
- Portions: 4 servings

Ingredients and quantity:
  - 1 tablespoon coconut oil
  - 1 onion, diced
  - 2 cloves garlic, minced
  - 1 tablespoon grated fresh ginger
  - 2 tablespoons Thai red curry paste
  - 4 cups vegetable broth
  - 1 can (14 oz) coconut milk
  - 2 cups diced vegetables
    (e.g., bell peppers, carrots, broccoli)
  - 1 cup cooked rice noodles or rice
  - 2 tablespoons soy sauce
  - 1 tablespoon lime juice
  - Salt and pepper to taste
  - Fresh cilantro, for garnish

Procedure:
  1. In a large pot, heat coconut oil over medium heat. Add diced onion, minced garlic,
     and grated ginger. Cook until softened.
  2. Stir in Thai red curry paste and cook for 1-2 minutes.
  3. Add vegetable broth and coconut milk to the pot. Bring to a simmer.
  4. Add diced vegetables and cooked rice noodles or rice. Cook until the vegetables
     are tender.
  5. Stir in soy sauce, lime juice, salt, and pepper.
  6. Adjust seasoning if necessary and serve hot, garnished with fresh cilantro.

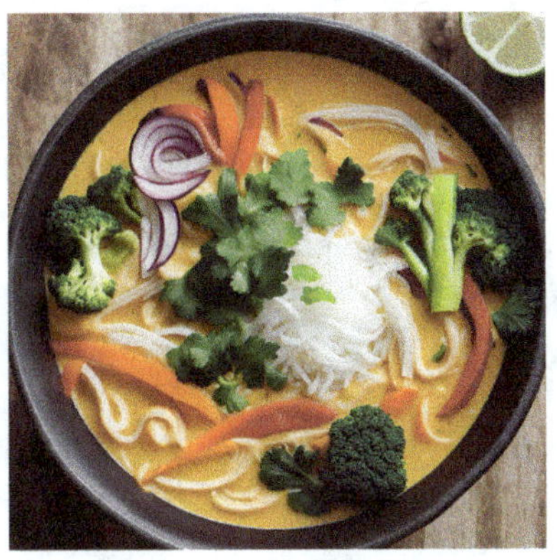

Nutritional values (per serving):
  - Calories: 280
  - Protein: 4g
  - Fat: 20g
  - Carbohydrates: 25g
  - Fiber: 3g

Shopping list:
- Coconut oil
- Onion
- Garlic
- Fresh ginger
- Thai red curry paste
- Vegetable broth
- Coconut milk
- Assorted vegetables (bell peppers,
  carrots, broccoli)
- Rice noodles or rice
- Soy sauce
- Lime
- Fresh cilantro

27. Mediterranean Chickpea Salad

- Preparation time: 15 minutes
- Cooking time: 0 minutes
- Portions: 4 servings

Ingredients and quantity:
- 2 cans (15 oz each) chickpeas, drained and rinsed
- 1 cucumber, diced
- 1 cup cherry tomatoes, halved
- 1/2 red onion, thinly sliced
- 1/4 cup chopped fresh parsley
- 1/4 cup chopped fresh mint
- 1/4 cup crumbled feta cheese (optional)
- 2 tablespoons extra virgin olive oil
- 2 tablespoons lemon juice
- 1 teaspoon dried oregano
- Salt and pepper to taste

Procedure:
1. In a large salad bowl, combine chickpeas, diced cucumber, halved cherry tomatoes, thinly sliced red onion, chopped fresh parsley, and chopped fresh mint.
2. If using, sprinkle crumbled feta cheese over the salad.
3. In a small bowl, whisk together extra virgin olive oil, lemon juice, dried oregano, salt, and pepper to make the dressing.
4. Pour the dressing over the chickpea salad and toss to coat evenly.
5. Serve immediately or refrigerate until ready to serve.

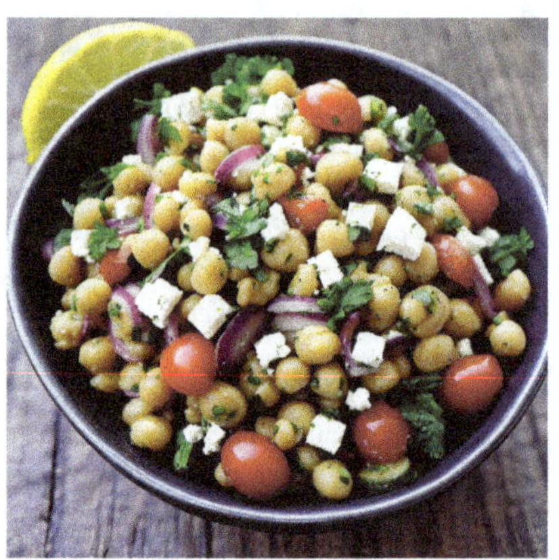

Nutritional values (per serving):
- Calories: 270
- Protein: 10g
- Fat: 10g
- Carbohydrates: 35g
- Fiber: 10g

Shopping list:
- Canned chickpeas
- Cucumber
- Cherry tomatoes
- Red onion
- Fresh parsley
- Fresh mint
- Feta cheese (optional)
- Extra virgin olive oil
- Lemon
- Dried oregano

28. Roasted Beet Salad with Goat Cheese

- Preparation time: 15 minutes
- Cooking time: 45 minutes
- Portions: 4 servings

Ingredients and quantity:
  - 4 medium beets, peeled and diced
- 2 tablespoons olive oil
- Salt and pepper to taste
- 4 cups mixed salad greens
- 1/2 cup crumbled goat cheese
- 1/4 cup chopped walnuts
- Balsamic vinegar, for drizzling

Procedure:
  1. Preheat the oven to 400°F (200°C). Line a baking sheet with parchment paper.
  2. In a bowl, toss diced beets with olive oil, salt, and pepper until evenly coated.
  3. Spread the seasoned beets on the prepared baking sheet in a single layer.
  4. Roast in the preheated oven for 40-45 minutes, or until the beets are tender and caramelized.
  5. Arrange mixed salad greens on serving plates. Top with roasted beets, crumbled goat cheese, and chopped walnuts.
  6. Drizzle balsamic vinegar over the salad and serve immediately.

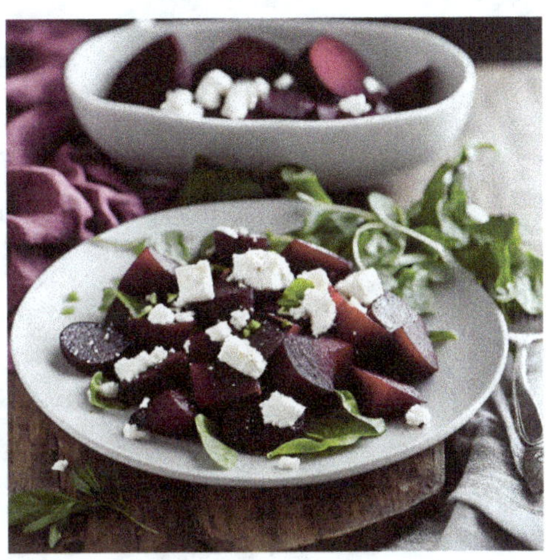

Nutritional values (per serving):
  - Calories: 220
  - Protein: 7g
  - Fat: 14g
  - Carbohydrates: 18g
  - Fiber: 5g

Shopping list:
  - Beets
  - Olive oil
  - Mixed salad greens
  - Goat cheese
  - Walnuts
  - Balsamic vinegar

29. Butternut Squash Soup with Sage

- Preparation time: 15 minutes
- Cooking time: 30 minutes
- Portions: 6 servings

Ingredients and quantity:
- 1 butternut squash, peeled, seeded, and diced
- 1 tablespoon olive oil
- 1 onion, diced
- 2 cloves garlic, minced
- 4 cups vegetable broth
- 1 teaspoon dried sage
- Salt and pepper to taste
- 1/4 cup coconut milk (optional)

Procedure:
1. In a large pot, heat olive oil over medium heat. Add diced onion and minced garlic. Cook until softened.
2. Add diced butternut squash, vegetable broth, dried sage, salt, and pepper to the pot. Bring to a boil.
3. Reduce heat to low and simmer for 20-25 minutes, or until the squash is tender.
4. Use an immersion blender to puree the soup until smooth. Alternatively, transfer the soup to a blender and blend until smooth, then return to the pot.
5. Stir in coconut milk (if using) and adjust seasoning if necessary.
6. Serve hot, garnished with fresh sage leaves if desired.

Nutritional values (per serving):
- Calories: 120
- Protein: 2g
- Fat: 4g
- Carbohydrates: 22g
- Fiber: 4g
- Shopping list:
- Butternut squash
- Olive oil
- Onion
- Garlic
- Vegetable broth
- Dried sage
- Coconut milk (optional)

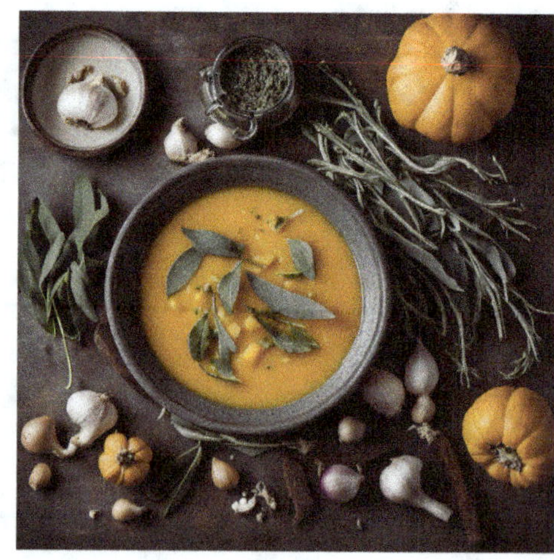

30. Greek Salad with Tofu Feta

- Preparation time: 15 minutes
- Cooking time: 0 minutes
- Portions: 4 servings

Ingredients and quantity:
- 1 block (14 oz) extra firm tofu, pressed and cubed
- 2 tablespoons lemon juice
- 1 tablespoon apple cider vinegar
- 1 tablespoon olive oil
- 1 teaspoon dried oregano
- 1/2 teaspoon garlic powder
- Salt and pepper to taste
- 1 cucumber, diced
- 1 bell pepper, diced
- 1 cup cherry tomatoes, halved
- 1/4 cup Kalamata olives, pitted
- 1/4 cup red onion, thinly sliced
- 1/4 cup fresh parsley, chopped
- 1/4 cup extra virgin olive oil
- 2 tablespoons red wine vinegar
- Salt and pepper to taste

Procedure:

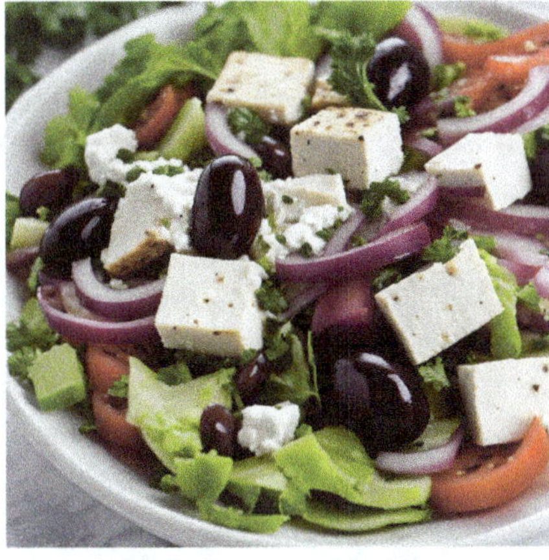

1. In a small bowl, whisk together lemon juice, apple cider vinegar, olive oil, dried oregano, garlic powder, salt, and pepper to make the marinade.
2. Place the cubed tofu in a shallow dish and pour the marinade over it. Toss gently to coat the tofu evenly. Allow it to marinate for at least 15 minutes.
3. In a large salad bowl, combine diced cucumber, bell pepper, cherry tomatoes, Kalamata olives, red onion, and fresh parsley.
4. In a small bowl, whisk together extra virgin olive oil, red wine vinegar, salt, and pepper to make the dressing.
5. Add the marinated tofu to the salad bowl and toss gently to combine.
6. Drizzle the dressing over the salad and toss again to coat everything evenly.
7. Serve immediately as a refreshing and nutritious meal.

Nutritional values (per serving):
- Calories: 280
- Protein: 12g
- Fat: 22g
- Carbohydrates: 14g
- Fiber: 4g

Shopping list:
- Extra firm tofu
- Lemon
- Apple cider vinegar
- Olive oil
- Dried oregano
- Garlic powder
- Cucumber
- Bell pepper
- Cherry tomatoes
- Kalamata olives
- Red onion
- Fresh parsley
- Red wine vinegar

Chapter 4

Main Dishes - Pasta and Grains

31. Spaghetti Aglio e Olio with Cherry Tomatoes

- Preparation time: 10 minutes
- Cooking time: 15 minutes
- Portions: 4 servings

Ingredients and quantity:
  - 12 oz spaghetti
  - 1/4 cup extra virgin olive oil
  - 4 cloves garlic, thinly sliced
  - 1/2 teaspoon red pepper flakes
  - 1 cup cherry tomatoes, halved
  - Salt and pepper to taste
  - Fresh parsley, chopped, for garnish

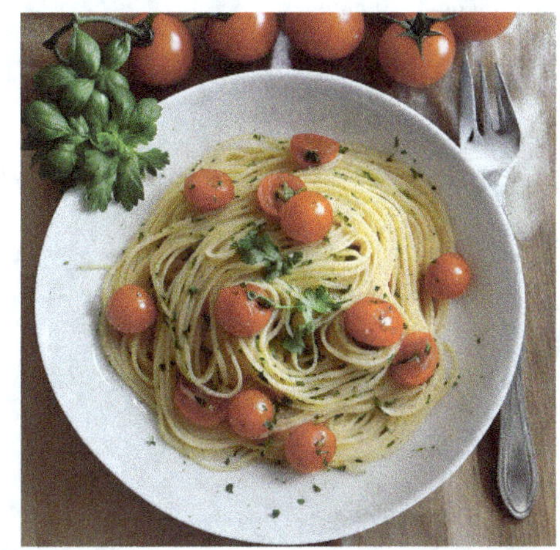

Procedure:
  1. Cook spaghetti according to package instructions until al dente. Drain and set aside.
  2. In a large skillet, heat olive oil over medium heat. Add sliced garlic and red pepper flakes. Cook until garlic is golden brown and fragrant.
  3. Add cherry tomatoes to the skillet and cook for 2-3 minutes, until they start to soften.
  4. Toss cooked spaghetti into the skillet with the garlic, oil, and tomatoes. Season with salt and pepper to taste. Cook for another 2-3 minutes, tossing to coat the spaghetti evenly.
  5. Serve hot, garnished with chopped fresh parsley.

Nutritional values (per serving):
  - Calories: 350
  - Protein: 8g
  - Fat: 14g
  - Carbohydrates: 50g
  - Fiber: 3g

Shopping list:
  - Spaghetti
  - Extra virgin olive oil
  - Garlic
  - Red pepper flakes
  - Cherry tomatoes
  - Fresh parsley

32. Vegan Pad Thai with Tofu

- Preparation time: 20 minutes
- Cooking time: 15 minutes
- Portions: 4 servings

Ingredients and quantity:
- 8 oz rice noodles
- 1 block (14 oz) extra firm tofu, pressed
  and cubed
- 2 tablespoons vegetable oil
- 2 cloves garlic, minced
- 1 red bell pepper, thinly sliced
- 1 carrot, julienned

- 2 cups bean sprouts
- 1/4 cup chopped peanuts
- 2 green onions, sliced
- Lime wedges, for serving
- Fresh cilantro, for garnish
- Pad Thai sauce:
  - 3 tablespoons soy sauce
  - 2 tablespoons maple syrup
  - 1 tablespoon rice vinegar
  - 1 tablespoon lime juice
  - 1 tablespoon sriracha sauce

Procedure:
1. Cook rice noodles according to package instructions until al dente. Drain and set aside.
2. In a small bowl, whisk together all the ingredients for the Pad Thai sauce.
3. In a large skillet or wok, heat vegetable oil over medium-high heat. Add minced garlic and cubed tofu. Cook until tofu is golden brown on all sides.
4. Add sliced red bell pepper and julienned carrot to the skillet. Stir-fry for 2-3 minutes until vegetables are tender-crisp.
5. Add cooked rice noodles and bean sprouts to the skillet. Pour the Pad Thai sauce over the noodles and vegetables. Toss everything together until well combined and heated through.
6. Serve hot, garnished with chopped peanuts, sliced green onions, lime wedges, and fresh cilantro.

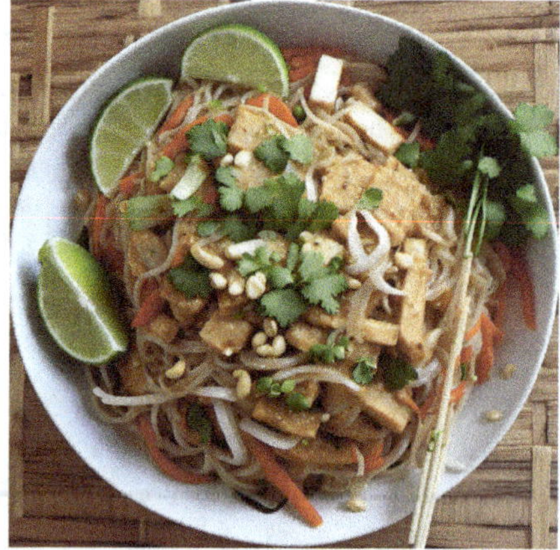

Nutritional values (per serving):
- Calories: 420
- Protein: 12g
- Fat: 15g
- Carbohydrates: 60g
- Fiber: 6g

Shopping list:
- Rice noodles
- Extra firm tofu
- Vegetable oil
- Garlic
- Red bell pepper
- Carrot
- Bean sprouts
- Peanuts
- Green onions
- Lime
- Fresh cilantro
- Soy sauce
- Maple syrup
- Rice vinegar
- Sriracha sauce

33. Mushroom Risotto with Arborio Rice

- Preparation time: 10 minutes
- Cooking time: 30 minutes
- Portions: 4 servings

Ingredients and quantity:
- 1 cup Arborio rice
- 4 cups vegetable broth
- 2 tablespoons olive oil
- 1 onion, finely chopped
- 2 cloves garlic, minced
- 8 oz mushrooms, sliced
- 1/4 cup dry white wine (optional)
- 1/4 cup grated Parmesan cheese
  (or nutritional yeast for a vegan option)
- Salt and pepper to taste
- Fresh parsley, chopped, for garnish

Procedure:

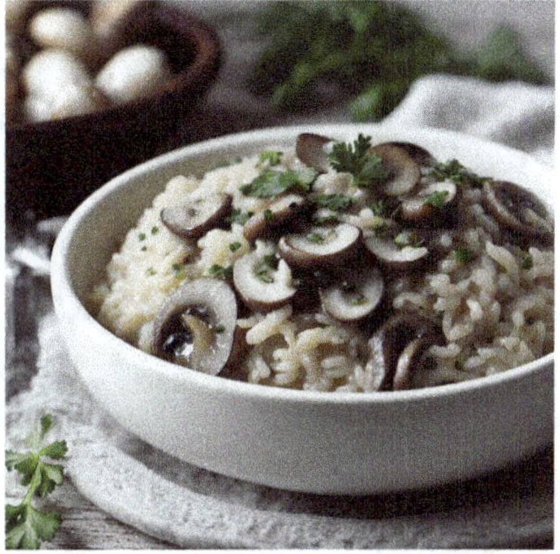

1. In a saucepan, heat the vegetable broth over low heat and keep it warm.
2. In a large skillet, heat olive oil over medium heat. Add chopped onion and minced garlic. Cook until softened, about 3-4 minutes.
3. Add sliced mushrooms to the skillet and cook until they release their juices and become golden brown.
4. Stir in Arborio rice and cook for 1-2 minutes, stirring constantly until the rice is well coated with oil.
5. If using, pour in the white wine and stir until it is absorbed by the rice.
6. Begin adding the warm vegetable broth, one ladleful at a time, stirring constantly and allowing each addition to be absorbed before adding more. Continue until the rice is creamy and tender but still slightly al dente, about 20-25 minutes.
7. Remove from heat and stir in grated Parmesan cheese (or nutritional yeast). Season with salt and pepper to taste.
8. Serve hot, garnished with chopped fresh parsley.

Nutritional values (per serving):
- Calories: 300
- Protein: 8g
- Fat: 8g
- Carbohydrates: 45g
- Fiber: 3g

Shopping list:
- Arborio rice
- Vegetable broth
- Olive oil
- Onion
- Garlic
- Mushrooms
- Dry white wine (optional)
- Parmesan cheese (or nutritional yeast)
- Fresh parsley

34. Quinoa Stuffed Peppers

- Preparation time: 15 minutes
- Cooking time: 40 minutes
- Portions: 4 servings

Ingredients and quantity:
- 4 large bell peppers, any color
- 1 cup quinoa, rinsed
- 2 cups vegetable broth
- 1 tablespoon olive oil
- 1 onion, chopped
- 2 cloves garlic, minced
- 1 can (14 oz) black beans, drained and rinsed
- 1 cup corn kernels (fresh or frozen)
- 1 teaspoon ground cumin
- 1/2 teaspoon chili powder
- Salt and pepper to taste
- 1/2 cup shredded cheese (cheddar, mozzarella, or vegan cheese for a dairy-free option)
- Fresh cilantro, chopped, for garnish

Procedure:
1. Preheat the oven to 375°F (190°C). Prepare a baking dish by lightly greasing it with olive oil.
2. Cut the tops off the bell peppers and remove the seeds and membranes. Place the peppers upright in the prepared baking dish.
3. In a saucepan, heat olive oil over medium heat. Add chopped onion and minced garlic. Cook until softened, about 3-4 minutes.
4. Add rinsed quinoa to the saucepan and toast for 1-2 minutes, stirring constantly.
5. Pour in the vegetable broth and bring to a boil. Reduce heat to low, cover, and simmer for 15-20 minutes until quinoa is cooked and liquid is absorbed.
6. In a large bowl, combine cooked quinoa, black beans, corn kernels, ground cumin, chili powder, salt, and pepper. Mix well.
7. Stuff each bell pepper with the quinoa mixture and place them back into the baking dish.
8. Cover the baking dish with aluminum foil and bake in the preheated oven for 25-30 minutes until the peppers are tender.
9. Remove the foil, sprinkle shredded cheese over the stuffed peppers, and bake for an additional 5 minutes until the cheese is melted and bubbly.
10. Serve hot, garnished with chopped fresh cilantro.

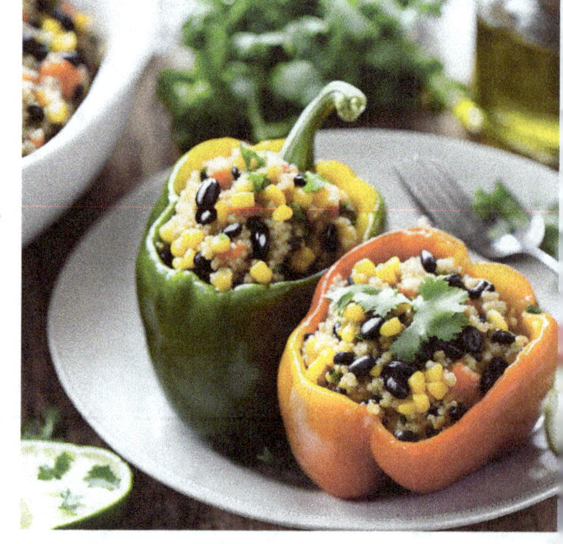

Nutritional values (per serving):
- Calories: 350
- Protein: 14g
- Fat: 8g
- Carbohydrates: 55g
- Fiber: 10g

Shopping list:
- Bell peppers
- Quinoa
- Vegetable broth
- Olive oil
- Onion
- Garlic
- Black beans
- Corn kernels
- Ground cumin
- Chili powder
- Shredded cheese (or vegan cheese)
- Fresh cilantro

35. Veggie Stir-Fry with Brown Rice

- Preparation time: 15 minutes
- Cooking time: 15 minutes
- Portions: 4 servings

Ingredients and quantity:
- 1 cup brown rice
- 2 cups water
- 2 tablespoons vegetable oil
- 1 onion, sliced
- 2 cloves garlic, minced
- 1 bell pepper, sliced
- 1 cup broccoli florets
- 1 carrot, julienned
- 1 cup snow peas
- 1 cup mushrooms, sliced
- 1/4 cup soy sauce
  (or tamari for a gluten-free option)
- 1 tablespoon rice vinegar
- 1 tablespoon maple syrup
- 1 teaspoon sesame oil
- 1 teaspoon cornstarch mixed with
  2 tablespoons water
- Sesame seeds, for garnish
- Green onions, sliced, for garnish

Procedure:
1. Cook brown rice according to package instructions until tender.
2. In a wok or large skillet, heat vegetable oil over medium-high heat. Add sliced onion and minced garlic. Stir-fry for 2-3 minutes until fragrant.
3. Add sliced bell pepper, broccoli florets, julienned carrot, snow peas, and sliced mushrooms to the wok. Stir-fry for 4-5 minutes until vegetables are tender-crisp.
4. In a small bowl, whisk together soy sauce, rice vinegar, maple syrup, sesame oil, and cornstarch mixture. Pour the sauce over the vegetables in the wok.
5. Cook for another 2-3 minutes, stirring constantly, until the sauce thickens and coats the vegetables.
6. Serve the stir-fried vegetables over cooked brown rice.
7. Garnish with sesame seeds and sliced green onions.

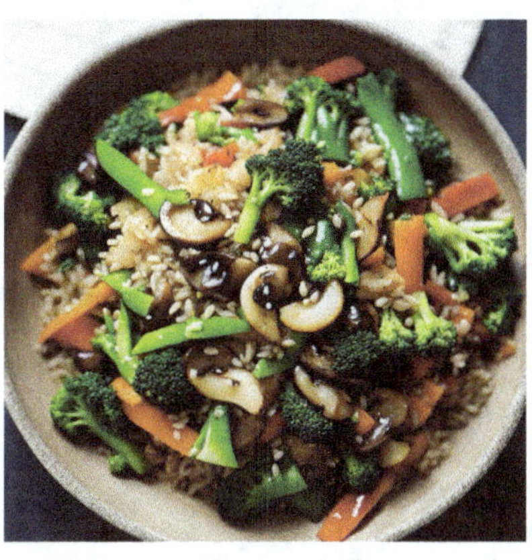

Nutritional values (per serving):
- Calories: 280
- Protein: 8g
- Fat: 7g
- Carbohydrates: 45g
- Fiber: 6g

Shopping list:
- Brown rice
- Vegetable oil
- Onion
- Garlic
- Bell pepper
- Broccoli
- Carrot
- Snow peas
- Mushrooms
- Soy sauce (or tamari)
- Rice vinegar
- Maple syrup
- Sesame oil
- Cornstarch
- Sesame seeds
- Green onions

36. Spinach and Ricotta Stuffed Shells

- Preparation time: 20 minutes
- Cooking time: 30 minutes
- Portions: 4 servings

Ingredients and quantity:
  - 16 jumbo pasta shells
  - 2 cups ricotta cheese
  - 1 cup chopped spinach, cooked and drained
  - 1/2 cup grated Parmesan cheese
  - 1 egg, beaten
  - 1 teaspoon dried basil
  - 1 teaspoon dried oregano
  - Salt and pepper to taste
  - 2 cups marinara sauce
  - Fresh basil leaves, for garnish

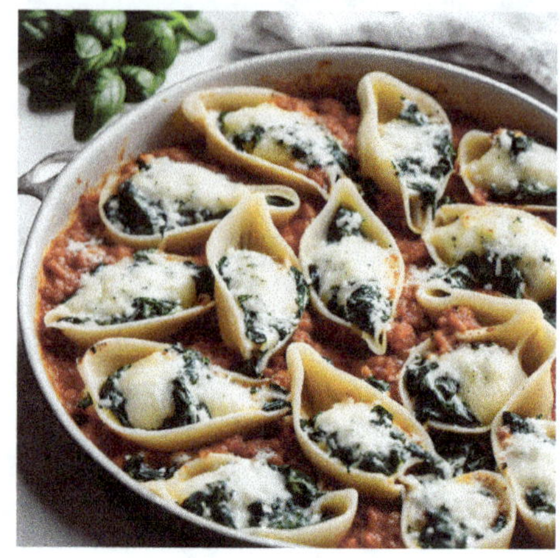

Procedure:
  1. Preheat the oven to 375°F (190°C). Lightly grease a baking dish with olive oil.
  2. Cook jumbo pasta shells according to package instructions until al dente. Drain and set aside.
  3. In a mixing bowl, combine ricotta cheese, cooked chopped spinach, grated Parmesan cheese, beaten egg, dried basil, dried oregano, salt, and pepper. Mix well.
  4. Stuff each cooked pasta shell with the spinach and ricotta mixture.
  5. Spread a thin layer of marinara sauce on the bottom of the prepared baking dish. Arrange the stuffed shells in the dish.
  6. Pour the remaining marinara sauce over the stuffed shells.
  7. Cover the baking dish with aluminum foil and bake in the preheated oven for 20 minutes.
  8. Remove the foil and bake for an additional 10 minutes until the sauce is bubbly and the shells are heated through.
  9. Serve hot, garnished with fresh basil leaves.

Nutritional values (per serving):
  - Calories: 380
  - Protein: 22g
  - Fat: 15g
  - Carbohydrates: 40g
  - Fiber: 4g

Shopping list:
- Jumbo pasta shells
- Ricotta cheese
- Spinach
- Parmesan cheese
- Egg
- Dried basil
- Dried oregano
- Marinara sauce
- Fresh basil leaves

37. Eggplant Parmesan with Marinara Sauce

- Preparation time: 20 minutes
- Cooking time: 40 minutes
- Portions: 4 servings

Ingredients and quantity:
  - 1 large eggplant, sliced into rounds
  - 1 cup all-purpose flour
  - 2 eggs, beaten
  - 1 cup breadcrumbs
  - 1/2 cup grated Parmesan cheese
  - 2 cups marinara sauce
  - 1 cup shredded mozzarella cheese
  - Fresh basil leaves, for garnish
  - Salt and pepper to taste

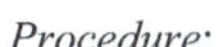

Procedure:
  1. Preheat the oven to 375°F (190°C). Line a
     baking sheet with parchment paper.
  2. Season eggplant slices with salt and let them sit for 10 minutes to release excess moisture. Pat dry
     with paper towels.
  3. Set up three shallow bowls: one with flour, one with beaten eggs, and one with breadcrumbs mixed
     with grated Parmesan cheese.
  4. Dredge each eggplant slice in flour, then dip in beaten eggs, and coat with breadcrumb mixture.
  5. Place breaded eggplant slices on the prepared baking sheet and bake in the preheated oven for 20
     minutes, flipping halfway through, until golden brown and crispy.
  6. Spread a thin layer of marinara sauce in the bottom of a baking dish. Arrange half of the baked
     eggplant slices in the dish.
  7. Top with half of the remaining marinara sauce and half of the shredded mozzarella cheese.
  8. Repeat with the remaining eggplant slices, marinara sauce, and mozzarella cheese.
  9. Bake in the oven for another 20 minutes until the cheese is melted and bubbly.
  10. Serve hot, garnished with fresh basil leaves.

Nutritional values (per serving):
  - Calories: 320
  - Protein: 15g
  - Fat: 12g
  - Carbohydrates: 40g
  - Fiber: 6g

Shopping list:
  - Eggplant
  - All-purpose flour
  - Eggs
  - Breadcrumbs
  - Parmesan cheese
  - Marinara sauce
  - Mozzarella cheese
  - Fresh basil leaves

38. Lemon Garlic Orzo with Asparagus

- Preparation time: 10 minutes
- Cooking time: 15 minutes
- Portions: 4 servings

Ingredients and quantity:
- 1 cup orzo pasta
- 1 bunch asparagus, trimmed and cut
  into bite-sized pieces
- 2 tablespoons olive oil
- 3 cloves garlic, minced
- Zest of 1 lemon
- Juice of 1 lemon
- 1/4 cup grated Parmesan cheese
  (optional)
- Salt and pepper to taste
- Fresh parsley, chopped, for garnish

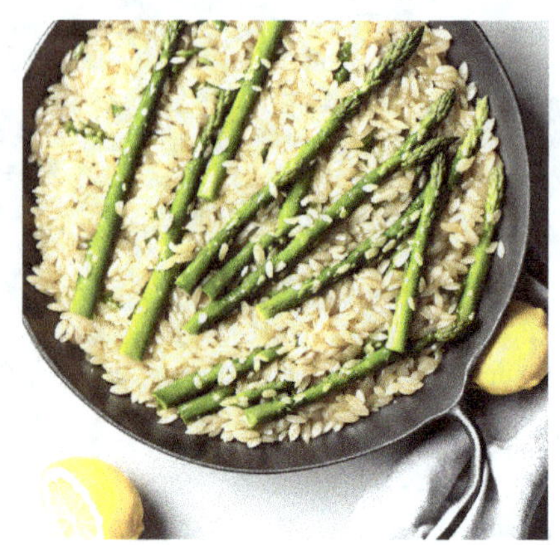

Procedure:
1. Cook orzo pasta according to package instructions until al dente. Drain and set aside.
2. In a large skillet, heat olive oil over medium heat. Add minced garlic and cook until
   fragrant, about 1 minute.
3. Add trimmed asparagus pieces to the skillet and sauté for 4-5 minutes until tender-crisp.
4. Add cooked orzo pasta to the skillet along with lemon zest and lemon juice.
   Toss to combine.
5. If using, stir in grated Parmesan cheese until melted and well incorporated.
6. Season with salt and pepper to taste.
7. Serve hot, garnished with chopped fresh parsley.

Nutritional values (per serving):
- Calories: 250
- Protein: 8g
- Fat: 7g
- Carbohydrates: 40g
- Fiber: 5g

Shopping list:
- Orzo pasta
- Asparagus
- Olive oil
- Garlic
- Lemon
- Parmesan cheese (optional)
- Fresh parsley

39. Vegan Chili with Kidney Beans

- Preparation time: 15 minutes
- Cooking time: 30 minutes
- Portions: 6 servings

Ingredients and quantity:
- 1 tablespoon olive oil
- 1 onion, chopped
- 3 cloves garlic, minced
- 1 bell pepper, diced
- 2 carrots, diced
- 2 celery stalks, diced
- 1 can (15 oz) kidney beans,
  drained and rinsed
- 1 can (15 oz) diced tomatoes
- 1 cup vegetable broth
- 2 tablespoons tomato paste
- 2 teaspoons chili powder
- 1 teaspoon ground cumin
- 1 teaspoon paprika
- Salt and pepper to taste
- Fresh cilantro, chopped, for garnish
- Avocado slices, for garnish

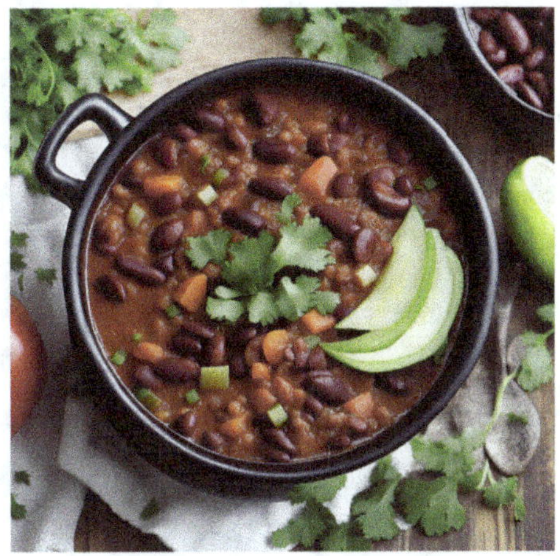

Procedure:
1. In a large pot, heat olive oil over medium heat. Add chopped onion and minced garlic. Cook until softened, about 3-4 minutes.
2. Add diced bell pepper, carrots, and celery to the pot. Cook for another 5 minutes until vegetables are tender.
3. Stir in drained and rinsed kidney beans, diced tomatoes, vegetable broth, tomato paste, chili powder, ground cumin, paprika, salt, and pepper.
4. Bring the chili to a simmer, then reduce heat to low. Cover and let it simmer for 20 minutes, stirring occasionally.
5. Taste and adjust seasoning if needed.
6. Serve hot, garnished with chopped fresh cilantro and avocado slices.

Nutritional values
  (per serving):
- Calories: 200
- Protein: 8g
- Fat: 4g
- Carbohydrates: 30g
- Fiber: 8g

Shopping list:
- Olive oil
- Onion
- Garlic
- Bell pepper
- Carrots
- Celery
- Kidney beans
- Diced tomatoes
- Vegetable broth
- Tomato paste
- Chili powder
- Ground cumin
- Paprika
- Fresh cilantro
- Avocado

40. Zucchini Noodles with Pesto

- Preparation time: 15 minutes
- Cooking time: 5 minutes
- Portions: 2 servings

Ingredients and quantity:
 - 2 medium zucchinis
 - 1 cup fresh basil leaves
 - 1/4 cup pine nuts
 - 2 cloves garlic, peeled
 - 1/4 cup grated Parmesan cheese
   (optional for non-vegan version)
 - 1/4 cup extra-virgin olive oil
 - Salt and pepper to taste
 - Cherry tomatoes, halved, for garnish
 - Fresh basil leaves, for garnish

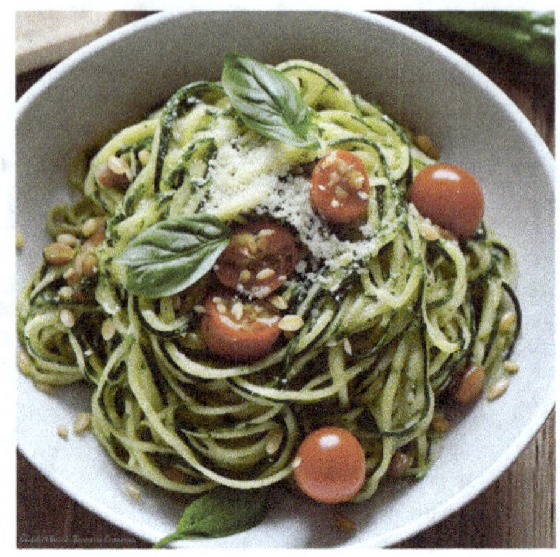

Procedure:
1. Using a spiralizer or vegetable peeler, create zucchini noodles from the zucchinis. Set aside.
2. In a food processor, combine fresh basil leaves, pine nuts, garlic cloves, and grated Parmesan cheese (if using). Pulse until ingredients are finely chopped.
3. With the food processor running, gradually pour in the extra-virgin olive oil until the mixture forms a smooth paste.
4. Season the pesto with salt and pepper to taste.
5. In a large skillet, heat a drizzle of olive oil over medium heat. Add zucchini noodles and sauté for 2-3 minutes until just tender.
6. Add the prepared pesto to the skillet with zucchini noodles. Toss until the noodles are evenly coated with pesto.
7. Cook for an additional 1-2 minutes, stirring constantly, until heated through.
8. Serve hot, garnished with halved cherry tomatoes and fresh basil leaves.

Nutritional values (per serving):
 - Calories: 250
 - Protein: 5g
 - Fat: 23g
 - Carbohydrates: 8g
 - Fiber: 3g

Shopping list:
 - Zucchinis
 - Fresh basil leaves
 - Pine nuts
 - Garlic
 - Parmesan cheese (optional)
 - Extra-virgin olive oil
 - Cherry tomatoes
 - Fresh basil leaves

Main Dishes - Protein Alternatives

41. Black Bean and Sweet Potato Tacos

- Preparation time: 15 minutes
- Cooking time: 25 minutes
- Portions: 4 servings

Ingredients and quantity:
  - 1 tablespoon olive oil
  - 1 onion, diced
  - 2 cloves garlic, minced
  - 1 sweet potato, peeled and diced
  - 1 can (15 oz) black beans,
    drained and rinsed
  - 1 teaspoon chili powder
  - 1/2 teaspoon ground cumin
  - Salt and pepper to taste
  - 8 small corn tortillas
  - Toppings: avocado slices, salsa,
    cilantro, lime wedges

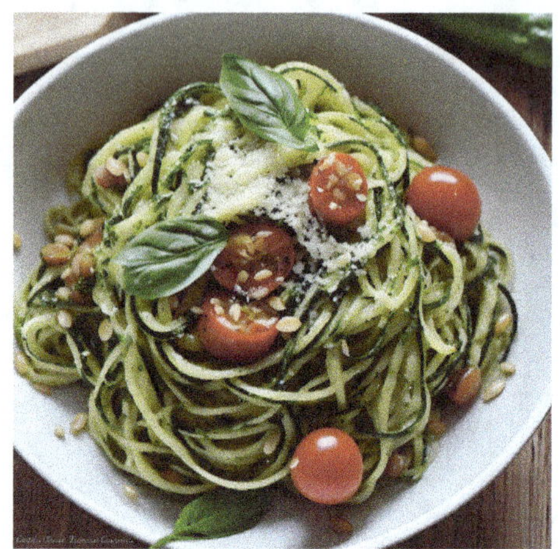

Procedure:
  1. Heat olive oil in a skillet over medium heat. Add diced onion and minced garlic,
     sauté until softened, about 3-4 minutes.
  2. Add diced sweet potato to the skillet and cook until tender, about 10-12 minutes.
  3. Stir in drained black beans, chili powder, ground cumin, salt, and pepper.
     Cook for an additional 5 minutes until heated through.
  4. Warm corn tortillas in a separate skillet or oven.
  5. Spoon the black bean and sweet potato mixture onto the warm tortillas.
  6. Serve hot, garnished with avocado slices, salsa, cilantro, and lime wedges.

Nutritional values (per serving):
  - Calories: 280
  - Protein: 8g
  - Fat: 5g
  - Carbohydrates: 52g
  - Fiber: 10g

Shopping list:
  - Olive oil
  - Onion
  - Garlic
  - Sweet potato
  - Black beans
  - Chili powder
  - Ground cumin
  - Corn tortillas
  - Avocado
  - Salsa
  - Cilantro
  - Lime

42. Lentil Shepherd's Pie

- Preparation time: 20 minutes
- Cooking time: 40 minutes
- Portions: 6 servings

Ingredients and quantity:
- 2 cups cooked lentils
- 2 tablespoons olive oil
- 1 onion, diced
- 2 carrots, diced
- 2 celery stalks, diced
- 2 cloves garlic, minced
- 1 cup frozen peas
- 1 cup vegetable broth
- 2 tablespoons tomato paste
- 1 teaspoon Worcestershire sauce (optional)
- Salt and pepper to taste
- 4 cups mashed potatoes

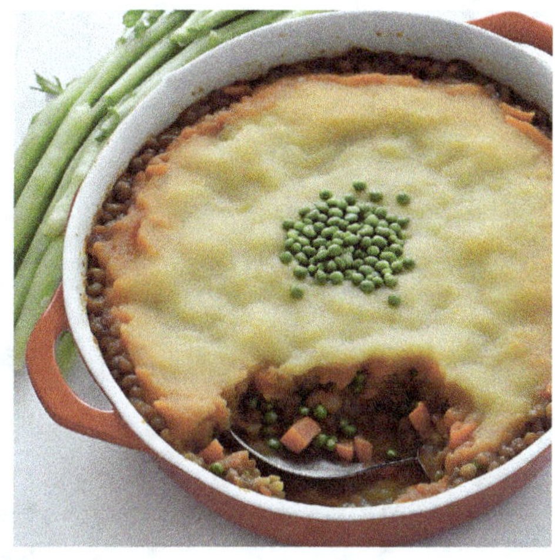

Procedure:
1. Preheat the oven to 375°F (190°C). Grease a baking dish.
2. Heat olive oil in a large skillet over medium heat. Add diced onion, carrots, celery, and minced garlic. Sauté until vegetables are softened, about 5-6 minutes.
3. Stir in cooked lentils, frozen peas, vegetable broth, tomato paste, Worcestershire sauce (if using), salt, and pepper. Cook for another 5 minutes until heated through.
4. Transfer the lentil mixture to the greased baking dish and spread it out evenly.
5. Spread mashed potatoes over the lentil mixture, creating an even layer.
6. Bake in the preheated oven for 25-30 minutes until the mashed potatoes are lightly golden on top.
7. Serve hot.

Nutritional values (per serving):
- Calories: 320
- Protein: 12g
- Fat: 8g
- Carbohydrates: 50g
- Fiber: 10g

Shopping list:
- Lentils
- Olive oil
- Onion
- Carrots
- Celery
- Garlic
- Frozen peas
- Vegetable broth
- Tomato paste
- Worcestershire sauce (optional)
- Potatoes

43. Tempeh Stir-Fry with Ginger-Sesame Sauce

- Preparation time: 15 minutes
- Cooking time: 20 minutes
- Portions: 4 servings

Ingredients and quantity:
  - 8 oz tempeh, sliced into strips
  - 2 tablespoons soy sauce
  - 1 tablespoon sesame oil
  - 1 tablespoon maple syrup
  - 2 cloves garlic, minced
  - 1 tablespoon fresh ginger, grated
  - 1 red bell pepper, sliced
  - 1 yellow bell pepper, sliced
  - 1 cup broccoli florets
  - 1 carrot, julienned
  - 2 green onions, chopped
  - Cooked brown rice or noodles,
    for serving
  - Sesame seeds, for garnish

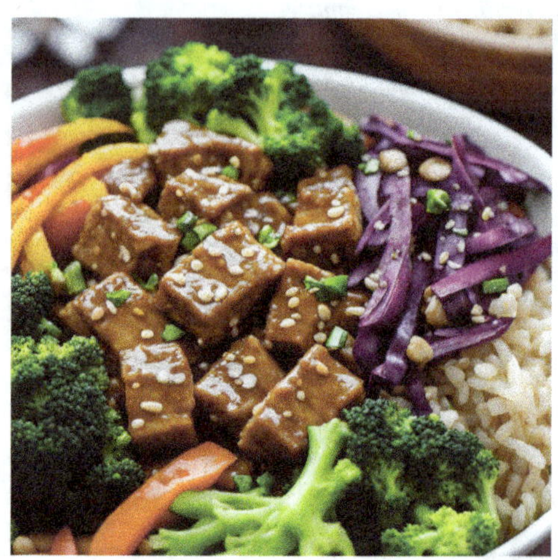

Procedure:
1. In a bowl, marinate tempeh strips in soy sauce, sesame oil, and maple syrup for 10 minutes.
2. In a large skillet or wok, heat some oil over medium-high heat. Add minced garlic and grated ginger, sauté until fragrant.
3. Add marinated tempeh to the skillet and cook until golden brown, about 3-4 minutes per side.
4. Add sliced bell peppers, broccoli florets, and julienned carrot to the skillet. Stir-fry for 5-6 minutes until vegetables are tender-crisp.
5. Pour in the prepared ginger-sesame sauce and toss to coat the tempeh and vegetables evenly.
6. Cook for another 2-3 minutes until the sauce thickens slightly.
7. Serve hot over cooked brown rice or noodles, garnished with chopped green onions and sesame seeds.

Nutritional values
(per serving):
  - Calories: 280
  - Protein: 18g
  - Fat: 10g
  - Carbohydrates: 32g
  - Fiber: 6g

Shopping list:
  - Tempeh
  - Soy sauce
  - Sesame oil
  - Maple syrup
  - Garlic
  - Fresh ginger
  - Red bell pepper
  - Yellow bell pepper
  - Broccoli florets
  - Carrot
  - Green onions
  - Brown rice or noodles
  - Sesame seeds

44. BBQ Jackfruit Sandwiches

- Preparation time: 15 minutes
- Cooking time: 30 minutes
- Portions: 4 servings

Ingredients and quantity:
  - 2 cans (20 oz each) young green jackfruit
    in brine, drained and rinsed
  - 1 tablespoon olive oil
  - 1 onion, diced
  - 2 cloves garlic, minced
  - 1 cup barbecue sauce
  - 4 hamburger buns
  - Coleslaw, for topping (optional)

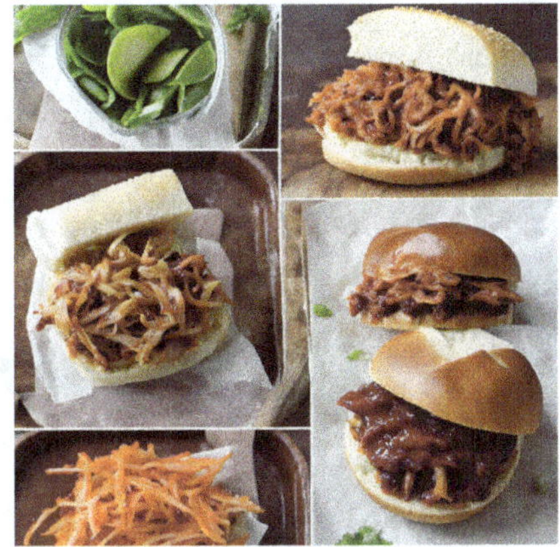

Procedure:
  1. Shred the drained and rinsed jackfruit using your hands or a fork to separate the fibers.
  2. In a skillet, heat olive oil over medium heat. Add diced onion and minced garlic,
     sauté until softened, about 3-4 minutes.
  3. Add shredded jackfruit to the skillet and cook for 5-6 minutes until slightly browned.
  4. Pour barbecue sauce over the jackfruit, stirring to coat evenly.
     Simmer for another 10-15 minutes until the sauce thickens and jackfruit is tender.
  5. Toast hamburger buns lightly.
  6. Spoon BBQ jackfruit mixture onto the bottom half of each hamburger bun.
  7. Top with coleslaw if desired, then cover with the top half of the bun.
  8. Serve hot.

Nutritional values (per serving):
  - Calories: 320
  - Protein: 4g
  - Fat: 6g
  - Carbohydrates: 65g
  - Fiber: 5g

Shopping list:
  - Canned young green jackfruit in brine
  - Olive oil
  - Onion
  - Garlic
  - Barbecue sauce
  - Hamburger buns
  - Coleslaw (optional)

45. Chickpea Tikka Masala

- Preparation time: 15 minutes
- Cooking time: 30 minutes
- Portions: 4 servings

Ingredients and quantity:
- 2 cans (15 oz each) chickpeas, drained and rinsed
- 1 tablespoon olive oil
- 1 onion, diced
- 2 cloves garlic, minced
- 1 tablespoon grated fresh ginger
- 1 can (14 oz) diced tomatoes
- 1/2 cup coconut milk
- 2 tablespoons tomato paste
- 2 teaspoons garam masala
- 1 teaspoon ground cumin
- 1 teaspoon ground coriander
- 1/2 teaspoon turmeric
- Salt and pepper to taste
- Fresh cilantro, for garnish
- Cooked rice, for serving

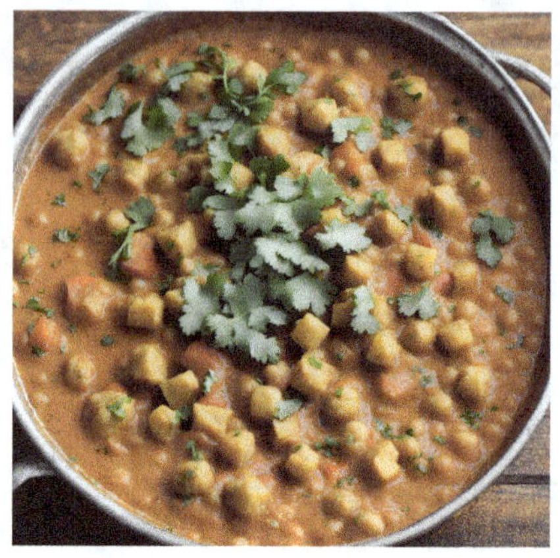

Procedure:
1. In a large skillet, heat olive oil over medium heat. Add diced onion, minced garlic, and grated ginger, sauté until softened, about 3-4 minutes.
2. Add diced tomatoes, coconut milk, tomato paste, garam masala, ground cumin, ground coriander, turmeric, salt, and pepper to the skillet. Stir to combine.
3. Simmer the sauce for 10-15 minutes until it thickens slightly.
4. Add drained and rinsed chickpeas to the skillet, stirring to coat with the sauce. Cook for an additional 10 minutes until heated through.
5. Serve hot over cooked rice, garnished with fresh cilantro.

Nutritional values
(per serving):
- Calories: 320
- Protein: 10g
- Fat: 12g
- Carbohydrates: 42g
- Fiber: 10g

Shopping list:
- Canned chickpeas
- Olive oil
- Onion
- Garlic
- Fresh ginger
- Canned diced tomatoes
- Coconut milk
- Tomato paste
- Garam masala
- Ground cumin
- Ground coriander
- Turmeric
- Fresh cilantro
- Rice

46. Tofu and Vegetable Stir-Fry with Peanut Sauce

- Preparation time: 15 minutes
- Cooking time: 15 minutes
- Portions: 4 servings

Ingredients and quantity:
  - 14 oz extra-firm tofu, drained
    and pressed, cut into cubes
  - 2 tablespoons soy sauce
  - 1 tablespoon sesame oil
  - 1 tablespoon maple syrup
  - 2 tablespoons peanut butter
  - 2 cloves garlic, minced
  - 1 tablespoon grated fresh ginger
  - 1 red bell pepper, sliced
  - 1 yellow bell pepper, sliced
  - 1 cup snap peas
  - 1 cup broccoli florets
  - Cooked brown rice, for serving
  - Chopped green onions and sesame seeds, for
    garnish

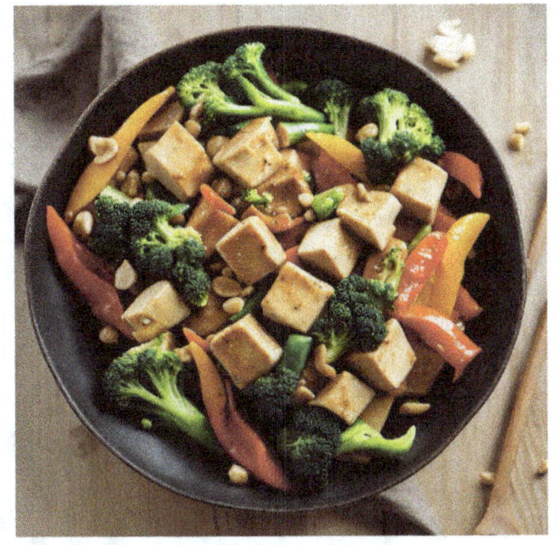

Procedure:
1. In a bowl, mix soy sauce, sesame oil, maple syrup, peanut butter, minced garlic, and grated
   ginger to make the peanut sauce.
2. In a large skillet or wok, heat some oil over medium-high heat. Add tofu cubes and cook until
   golden brown on all sides.
3. Add sliced bell peppers, snap peas, and broccoli florets to the skillet. Stir-fry for 3-4 minutes
   until vegetables are tender-crisp.
4. Pour the prepared peanut sauce over the tofu and vegetables. Stir well to coat evenly.
5. Cook for another 2-3 minutes until the sauce thickens slightly.
6. Serve hot over cooked brown rice, garnished with chopped green onions and sesame seeds.

Nutritional values
(per serving):
  - Calories: 280
  - Protein: 15g
  - Fat: 12g
  - Carbohydrates: 30g
  - Fiber: 6g

Shopping list:
- Extra-firm tofu
- Soy sauce
- Sesame oil
- Maple syrup
- Peanut butter
- Garlic
- Fresh ginger
- Red bell pepper
- Yellow bell pepper
- Snap peas
- Broccoli florets
- Brown rice
- Green onions
- Sesame seeds

47. Quinoa and Black Bean Enchiladas

- Preparation time: 20 minutes
- Cooking time: 30 minutes
- Portions: 4 servings

Ingredients and quantity:
- 1 cup quinoa, cooked
- 1 can (15 oz) black beans,
  drained and rinsed
- 1 cup corn kernels
- 1 red bell pepper, diced
- 1 onion, diced
- 2 cloves garlic, minced
- 1 teaspoon chili powder
- 1/2 teaspoon ground cumin
- 1/2 teaspoon paprika
- Salt and pepper to taste
- 8 small corn tortillas
- 1 can (10 oz) enchilada sauce
- 1 cup shredded vegan cheese
- Fresh cilantro, for garnish

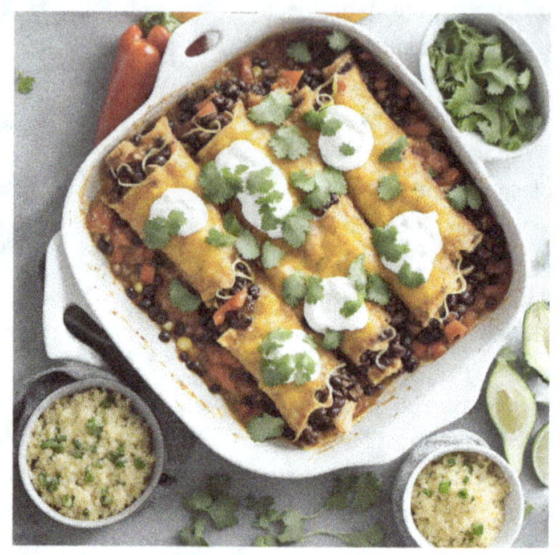

Procedure:
1. Preheat the oven to 375°F (190°C). Grease a baking dish.
2. In a large skillet, sauté diced onion and minced garlic until softened, about 3-4 minutes.
3. Add cooked quinoa, black beans, corn kernels, diced red bell pepper, chili powder, ground cumin, paprika, salt, and pepper to the skillet. Stir to combine and cook for another 5 minutes.
4. Warm corn tortillas in the microwave or oven until soft.
5. Spoon the quinoa and black bean mixture onto each tortilla, roll up, and place seam side down in the prepared baking dish.
6. Pour enchilada sauce over the rolled tortillas and sprinkle with shredded vegan cheese.
7. Bake in the preheated oven for 20 minutes until the cheese is melted and bubbly.
8. Serve hot, garnished with fresh cilantro.

Nutritional values (per serving):
- Calories: 380
- Protein: 15g
- Fat: 10g
- Carbohydrates: 60g
- Fiber: 12g

Shopping list:
- Quinoa
- Black beans
- Corn kernels
- Red bell pepper
- Onion
- Garlic
- Chili powder
- Ground cumin
- Paprika
- Corn tortillas
- Enchilada sauce
- Vegan cheese
- Fresh cilantr

48. Portobello Mushroom Burgers with Avocado

- Preparation time: 15 minutes
- Cooking time: 15 minutes
- Portions: 4 servings

Ingredients and quantity:
  - 4 large portobello mushrooms,
    stems removed
  - 2 tablespoons balsamic vinegar
  - 2 tablespoons olive oil
  - Salt and pepper to taste
  - 4 whole grain burger buns
  - 1 avocado, sliced
  - Lettuce leaves, tomato slices, red onion
    slices, for topping

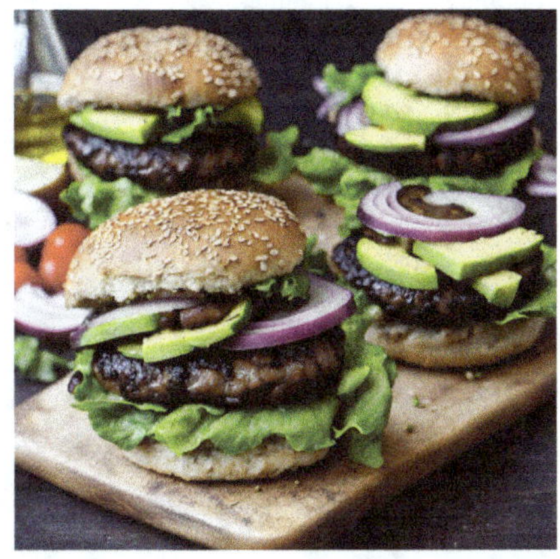

Procedure:
1. In a shallow dish, whisk together balsamic vinegar, olive oil, salt, and pepper. Place portobello mushrooms in the marinade, turning to coat evenly. Let marinate for 10 minutes.
2. Preheat grill or grill pan over medium heat. Remove mushrooms from the marinade and grill for 4-5 minutes per side until tender, brushing with additional marinade as needed.
3. Toast burger buns lightly on the grill.
4. Assemble the burgers by placing grilled portobello mushrooms on the bottom half of each burger bun.
5. Top with sliced avocado, lettuce leaves, tomato slices, and red onion slices.
6. Cover with the top half of the bun and serve immediately.

Nutritional values (per serving):
  - Calories: 250
  - Protein: 8g
  - Fat: 12g
  - Carbohydrates: 30g
  - Fiber: 6g

Shopping list:
  - Portobello mushrooms
  - Balsamic vinegar
  - Olive oil
  - Whole grain burger buns
  - Avocado
  - Lettuce leaves
  - Tomato
  - Red onion

49. Vegan Sloppy Joes with Lentils

- Preparation time: 15 minutes
- Cooking time: 30 minutes
- Portions: 4 servings

Ingredients and quantity:
- 1 cup dry brown lentils, rinsed
- 2 cups vegetable broth
- 1 tablespoon olive oil
- 1 onion, diced
- 2 cloves garlic, minced
- 1 red bell pepper, diced
- 1 carrot, grated
- 1 can (14 oz) crushed tomatoes
- 2 tablespoons tomato paste
- 2 tablespoons maple syrup
- 1 tablespoon soy sauce
- 1 tablespoon apple cider vinegar
- 1 teaspoon chili powder
- 1/2 teaspoon smoked paprika
- Salt and pepper to taste
- 4 whole grain hamburger buns
- Pickles and sliced red onion, for topping
  (optional)

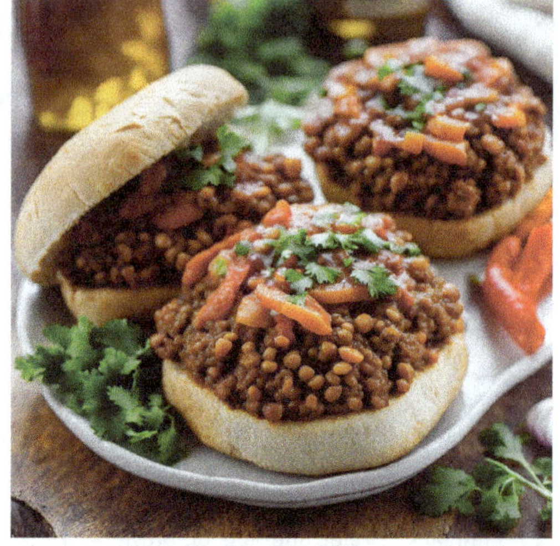

Procedure:
1. In a saucepan, combine the rinsed lentils and vegetable broth. Bring to a boil, then reduce heat, cover, and simmer for 20-25 minutes until lentils are tender and most of the liquid is absorbed.
2. In a large skillet, heat olive oil over medium heat. Add diced onion, minced garlic, diced red bell pepper, and grated carrot. Sauté until vegetables are softened, about 5-7 minutes.
3. Stir in the cooked lentils, crushed tomatoes, tomato paste, maple syrup, soy sauce, apple cider vinegar, chili powder, smoked paprika, salt, and pepper. Cook for an additional 5-10 minutes until heated through and flavors are well combined.
4. Toast the whole grain hamburger buns lightly.
5. Spoon the lentil mixture onto the bottom half of each hamburger bun. Top with pickles and sliced red onion if desired. Cover with the top half of the bun and serve immediately.

Nutritional values
(per serving):
- Calories: 350
- Protein: 15g
- Fat: 5g
- Carbohydrates: 65g
- Fiber: 15g

Shopping list:
- Maple syrup
- Soy sauce
- Apple cider vinegar
- Chili powder
- Smoked paprika
- Dry brown lentils
- Vegetable broth
- Olive oil
- Onion
- Garlic
- Red bell pepper
- Carrot
- Crushed tomatoes
- Tomato paste
- Whole grain
  hamburger buns
- Pickles
- Red onion

50. Cauliflower Steak with Chimichurri Sauce

- Preparation time: 10 minutes
- Cooking time: 25 minutes
- Portions: 4 servings

Ingredients and quantity:
  - 1 large head cauliflower
  - 2 tablespoons olive oil
  - Salt and pepper to taste
  - Chimichurri sauce:
    - 1 cup fresh parsley leaves, chopped
    - 1/4 cup fresh cilantro leaves, chopped
    - 2 cloves garlic, minced
    - 2 tablespoons red wine vinegar
    - 1/4 cup olive oil
    - 1/2 teaspoon red pepper flakes
    - Salt and pepper to taste

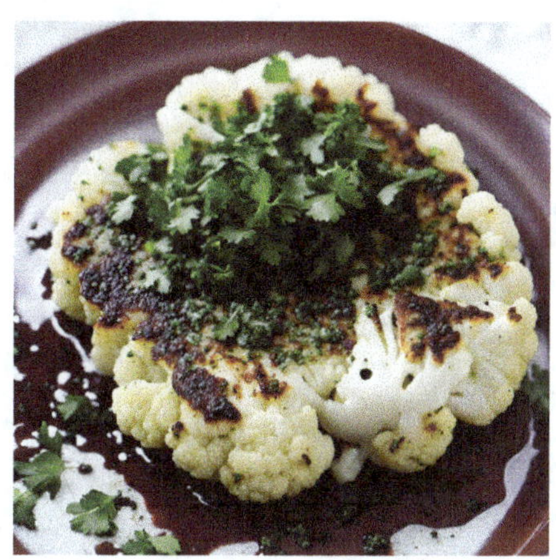

Procedure:
1. Preheat the oven to 400°F (200°C). Line a baking sheet with parchment paper.
2. Trim the leaves and stem of the cauliflower, leaving the core intact. Slice the cauliflower into 1-inch thick steaks.
3. Place cauliflower steaks on the prepared baking sheet. Brush both sides with olive oil and season with salt and pepper.
4. Roast in the preheated oven for 20-25 minutes, flipping halfway through, until the cauliflower is golden brown and tender.
5. While the cauliflower is roasting, prepare the chimichurri sauce. In a bowl, combine chopped parsley, chopped cilantro, minced garlic, red wine vinegar, olive oil, red pepper flakes, salt, and pepper. Stir well to combine.
6. Serve roasted cauliflower steaks hot, drizzled with chimichurri sauce.

Nutritional values (per serving):
- Calories: 150
- Protein: 5g
- Fat: 12g
- Carbohydrates: 10g
- Fiber: 5g

Shopping list:
- 1 large head cauliflower
- Olive oil
- Salt
- Pepper
- Fresh parsley
- Fresh cilantro
- Garlic
- Red wine vinegar
- Red pepper flakes

Sides and Accompaniments

51. Garlic Roasted Brussels Sprouts

- Preparation time: 10 minutes
- Cooking time: 25 minutes
- Portions: 4 servings

Ingredients and quantity:
  - 1 lb Brussels sprouts,
    trimmed and halved
  - 2 tablespoons olive oil
  - 3 cloves garlic, minced
  - Salt and pepper to taste

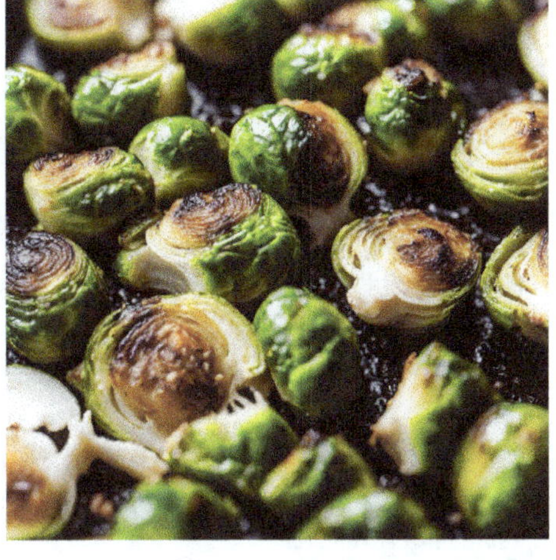

Procedure:
1. Preheat the oven to 400°F (200°C).
2. In a large bowl, toss Brussels sprouts with
   olive oil, minced garlic, salt, and pepper until
   evenly coated.
3. Spread Brussels sprouts in a single layer on a
   baking sheet lined with parchment paper.
4. Roast in the preheated oven for 20-25 minutes, stirring halfway through, until Brussels sprouts
   are tender and caramelized.
5. Serve hot as a delicious side dish.

Nutritional values (per serving):
  - Calories: 100
  - Protein: 4g
  - Fat: 7g
  - Carbohydrates: 10g
  - Fiber: 4g

Shopping list:
  - Brussels sprouts
  - Olive oil
  - Garlic
  - Salt
  - Pepper

52. Quinoa Pilaf with Herbs

- Preparation time: 15 minutes
- Cooking time: 20 minutes
- Portions: 4 servings

Ingredients and quantity:
  - 1 cup quinoa, rinsed
  - 2 cups vegetable broth
  - 1 tablespoon olive oil
  - 1 onion, diced
  - 2 cloves garlic, minced
  - 1 teaspoon dried thyme
  - 1 teaspoon dried oregano
  - Salt and pepper to taste
  - Fresh parsley, chopped, for garnish

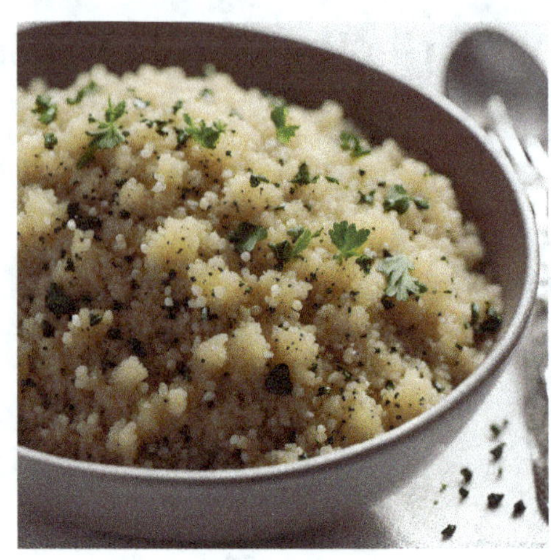

Procedure:

1. In a saucepan, bring vegetable broth to a boil. Add quinoa, reduce heat, cover, and simmer for 15-20 minutes until quinoa is cooked and liquid is absorbed.
2. In a separate skillet, heat olive oil over medium heat. Add diced onion and minced garlic, and sauté until softened.
3. Stir in cooked quinoa, dried thyme, dried oregano, salt, and pepper. Cook for an additional 2-3 minutes to allow flavors to meld.
4. Garnish with chopped fresh parsley before serving.

Nutritional values (per serving):
  - Calories: 200
  - Protein: 5g
  - Fat: 4g
  - Carbohydrates: 35g
  - Fiber: 5g

Shopping list:
  - Quinoa
  - Vegetable broth
  - Olive oil
  - Onion
  - Garlic
  - Dried thyme
  - Dried oregano
  - Salt
  - Pepper
  - Fresh parsley

53. Balsamic Glazed Carrots

- Preparation time: 10 minutes
- Cooking time: 20 minutes
- Portions: 4 servings

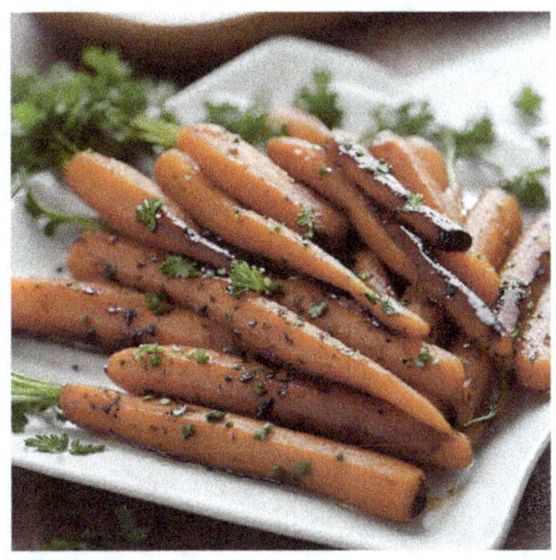

Ingredients and quantity:
- 1 lb carrots, peeled and sliced into sticks
- 2 tablespoons balsamic vinegar
- 1 tablespoon olive oil
- 1 tablespoon honey or maple syrup
- Salt and pepper to taste
- Fresh parsley, chopped, for garnish

Procedure:
1. Preheat the oven to 400°F (200°C).
2. In a bowl, toss carrot sticks with balsamic vinegar, olive oil, honey or maple syrup, salt, and pepper until evenly coated.
3. Spread carrots in a single layer on a baking sheet lined with parchment paper.
4. Roast in the preheated oven for 15-20 minutes, stirring halfway through, until carrots are tender and caramelized.
5. Garnish with chopped fresh parsley before serving.

Nutritional values (per serving):
- Calories: 80
- Protein: 1g
- Fat: 3g
- Carbohydrates: 14g
- Fiber: 3g

Shopping list:
- Carrots
- Balsamic vinegar
- Olive oil
- Honey or maple syrup
- Salt
- Pepper
- Fresh parsley

54. Grilled Asparagus with Lemon Zest

- Preparation time: 5 minutes
- Cooking time: 10 minutes
- Portions: 4 servings

Ingredients and quantity:
  - 1 lb asparagus spears, trimmed
  - 2 tablespoons olive oil
  - Zest of 1 lemon
  - Salt and pepper to taste

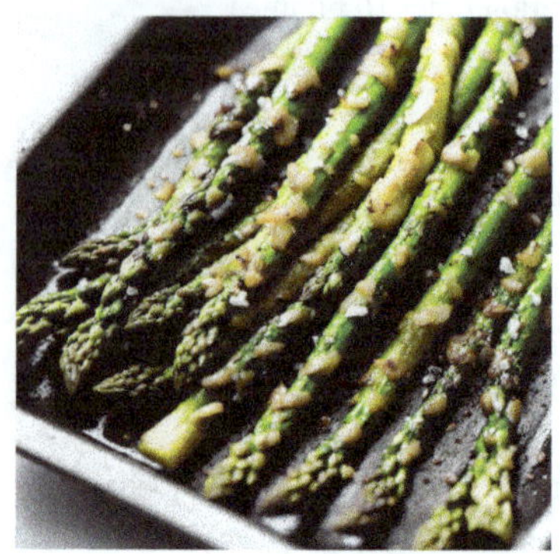

Procedure:
1. Preheat the grill to medium-high heat.
2. In a bowl, toss asparagus spears with olive oil
   until evenly coated.
3. Place asparagus on the preheated grill and cook for 5-7 minutes, turning occasionally, until tender and lightly charred.
4. Remove grilled asparagus from the grill and transfer to a serving platter.
5. Sprinkle lemon zest over the grilled asparagus and season with salt and pepper to taste.
6. Serve hot as a delightful side dish.

Nutritional values (per serving):
  - Calories: 60
  - Protein: 2g
  - Fat: 4g
  - Carbohydrates: 5g
  - Fiber: 3g

Shopping list:
  - Asparagus spears
  - Olive oil
  - Lemon
  - Salt
  - Pepper

55. Mashed Cauliflower with Vegan Butter

- Preparation time: 10 minutes
- Cooking time: 15 minutes
- Portions: 4 servings

Ingredients and quantity:
  - 1 head cauliflower, chopped into florets
  - 2 tablespoons vegan butter
  - Salt and pepper to taste
  - Chopped chives, for garnish (optional)

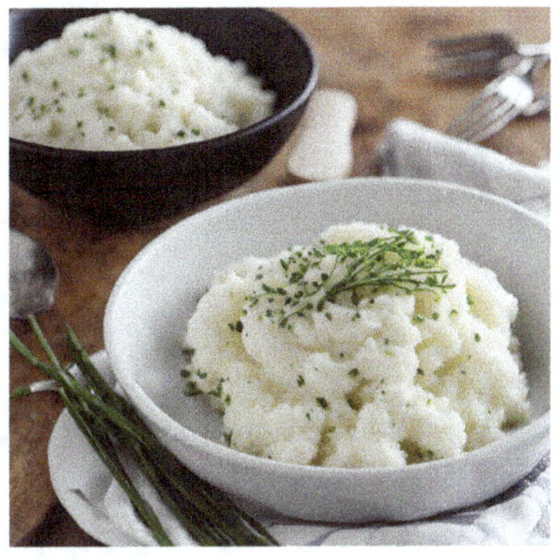

Procedure:
1. Bring a large pot of water to a boil. Add cauliflower
   florets and cook for 8-10 minutes until tender.
2. Drain cauliflower and transfer to a large bowl.
3. Add vegan butter to the bowl and mash cauliflower
   using a potato masher or fork until smooth.
4. Season with salt and pepper to taste and mix well.
5. Garnish with chopped chives if desired before serving.

Nutritional values (per serving):
  - Calories: 50
  - Protein: 2g
  - Fat: 3g
  - Carbohydrates: 5g
  - Fiber: 3g

Shopping list:
  - Cauliflower
  - Vegan butter
  - Salt
  - Pepper
  - Chopped chives (optional)

56. Roasted Sweet Potatoes with Rosemary

- Preparation time: 10 minutes
- Cooking time: 25 minutes
- Portions: 4 servings

Ingredients and quantity:
  - 2 large sweet potatoes,
    peeled and cubed
  - 2 tablespoons olive oil
  - 2 teaspoons chopped
    fresh rosemary
  - Salt and pepper to taste

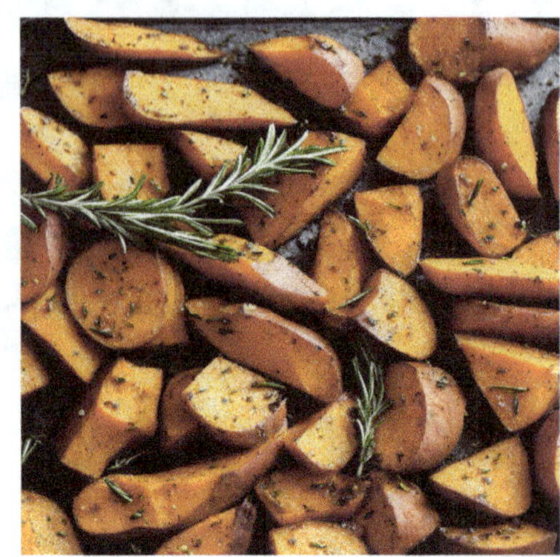

Procedure:
1. Preheat the oven to 400°F (200°C).
2. In a bowl, toss sweet potato cubes with olive oil, chopped fresh rosemary, salt, and pepper until evenly coated.
3. Spread sweet potatoes in a single layer on a baking sheet lined with parchment paper.
4. Roast in the preheated oven for 20-25 minutes, stirring halfway through, until sweet potatoes are tender and caramelized.
5. Serve hot as a delectable side dish.

Nutritional values (per serving):
  - Calories: 120
  - Protein: 2g
  - Fat: 5g
  - Carbohydrates: 18g
  - Fiber: 3g

Shopping list:
- Sweet potatoes
- Olive oil
- Fresh rosemary
- Salt
- Pepper

57. Sauteed Green Beans with Almonds

- Preparation time: 10 minutes
- Cooking time: 10 minutes
- Portions: 4 servings

Ingredients and quantity:
 - 1 lb green beans, trimmed
 - 2 tablespoons olive oil
 - 1/4 cup sliced almonds
 - 2 cloves garlic, minced
 - Salt and pepper to taste

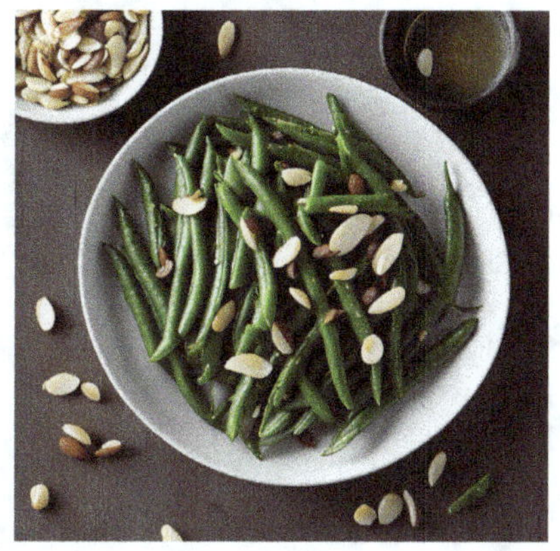

Procedure:
1. Heat olive oil in a large skillet over medium heat.
2. Add sliced almonds to the skillet and toast until lightly golden, about 2-3 minutes.
3. Add minced garlic to the skillet and sauté for 1 minute until fragrant.
4. Add trimmed green beans to the skillet and cook, stirring occasionally, for 5-7 minutes until green beans are tender-crisp.
5. Season with salt and pepper to taste and mix well.
6. Serve hot as a delightful side dish.

Nutritional values (per serving):
 - Calories: 80
 - Protein: 2g
 - Fat: 6g
 - Carbohydrates: 6g
 - Fiber: 3g

Shopping list:
- Green beans
- Olive oil
- Sliced almonds
- Garlic
- Salt
- Pepper

58. Lemon Herb Couscous

- Preparation time: 10 minutes
- Cooking time: 10 minutes
- Portions: 4 servings

Ingredients and quantity:
- 1 cup couscous
- 1 1/4 cups vegetable broth
- Zest of 1 lemon
- 2 tablespoons lemon juice
- 2 tablespoons chopped fresh herbs
  (such as parsley, mint, or basil)
- Salt and pepper to taste

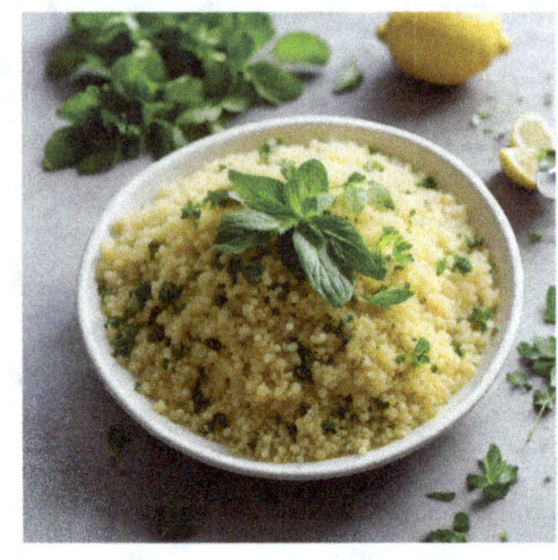

Procedure:
1. In a saucepan, bring vegetable broth to a boil.
2. Stir in couscous, cover, and remove from heat. Let it sit for 5 minutes.
3. Fluff couscous with a fork, then add lemon zest, lemon juice, chopped fresh herbs, salt, and pepper. Mix well.
4. Serve hot as a flavorful side dish.

Nutritional values (per serving):
- Calories: 200
- Protein: 5g
- Fat: 1g
- Carbohydrates: 40g
- Fiber: 3g

Shopping list:
- Couscous
- Vegetable broth
- Lemon
- Fresh herbs (parsley, mint, basil)
- Salt
- Pepper

59. Stuffed Bell Peppers with Quinoa and Vegetables

- Preparation time: 15 minutes
- Cooking time: 35 minutes
- Portions: 4 servings

Ingredients and quantity:
  - 4 bell peppers, any color, halved and seeds
    removed
  - 1 cup cooked quinoa
  - 1 cup diced mixed vegetables
    (such as onion, zucchini, carrot, and tomato)
  - 1/2 cup black beans, drained and rinsed
  - 1/2 cup corn kernels
  - 1 teaspoon olive oil
  - 1 teaspoon cumin
  - 1/2 teaspoon chili powder
  - Salt and pepper to taste
  - Chopped fresh cilantro, for garnish

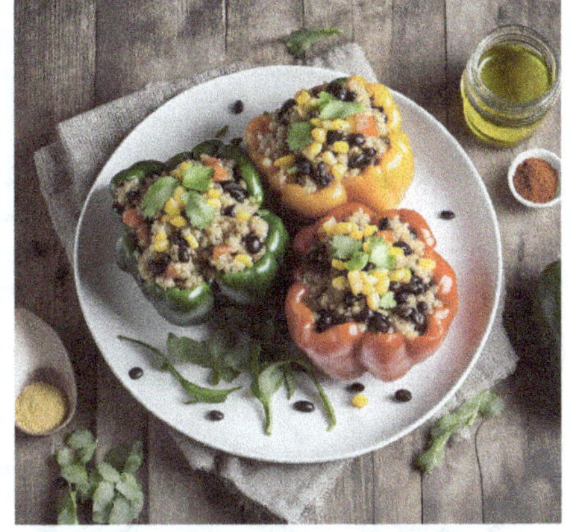

Procedure:
1. Preheat the oven to 375°F (190°C).
2. In a skillet, heat olive oil over medium heat. Add diced mixed vegetables and sauté until tender.
3. Stir in cooked quinoa, black beans, corn kernels, cumin, chili powder, salt, and pepper. Cook for
   an additional 2-3 minutes until well combined.
4. Fill each bell pepper half with the quinoa and vegetable mixture.
5. Place stuffed bell peppers on a baking dish and bake in the preheated oven for 25-30 minutes until
   peppers are tender.
6. Garnish with chopped fresh cilantro before serving.

Nutritional values (per serving):
  - Calories: 200
  - Protein: 7g
  - Fat: 2g
  - Carbohydrates: 40g
  - Fiber: 7g

Shopping list:
  - Bell peppers
  - Quinoa
  - Mixed vegetables
    (onion, zucchini, carrot, tomato)
  - Black beans
  - Corn kernels
  - Olive oil
  - Cumin
  - Chili powder
  - Salt
  - Pepper
  - Fresh cilantro

60. Vegan Cornbread with Maple Butter

- Preparation time: 15 minutes
- Cooking time: 25 minutes
- Portions: 9 servings

Ingredients and quantity:
  - 1 cup cornmeal
  - 1 cup all-purpose flour
  - 1/4 cup granulated sugar
  - 1 tablespoon baking powder
  - 1/2 teaspoon salt
  - 1 cup almond milk
    (or any plant-based milk)
  - 1/4 cup vegetable oil
  - 1/4 cup maple syrup
  - Vegan butter, for serving

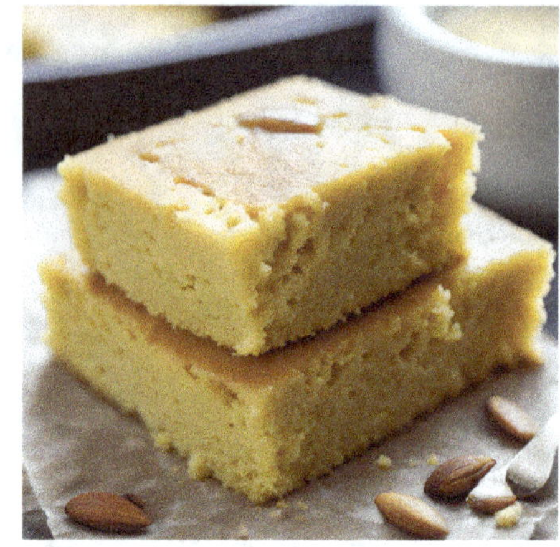

Procedure:
  1. Preheat the oven to 400°F (200°C). Grease an 8x8 inch baking pan.
  2. In a large bowl, whisk together cornmeal, flour, sugar, baking powder, and salt.
  3. In a separate bowl, mix almond milk, vegetable oil, and maple syrup.
  4. Pour the wet ingredients into the dry ingredients and stir until just combined. Do not overmix.
  5. Pour the batter into the prepared baking pan and smooth the top.
  6. Bake in the preheated oven for 20-25 minutes or until a toothpick inserted into the center comes out clean.
  7. Let the cornbread cool slightly before slicing. Serve warm with vegan butter and maple syrup.

Nutritional values (per serving):
  - Calories: 200
  - Protein: 2g
  - Fat: 8g
  - Carbohydrates: 30g
  - Fiber: 1g

Shopping list:
  - Cornmeal
  - All-purpose flour
  - Granulated sugar
  - Baking powder
  - Salt
  - Almond milk
    (or any plant-based milk)

Chapter 7

Light Meals and Bowls

61. Buddha Bowl with Quinoa, Avocado, and Chickpeas

- Preparation time: 15 minutes
- Cooking time: 20 minutes
- Portions: 2 servings

Ingredients and quantity:
  - 1 cup cooked quinoa
  - 1 ripe avocado, sliced
  - 1 cup cooked chickpeas
  - 1 cup mixed greens
  - 1 carrot, grated
  - 1/2 cucumber, sliced
  - 1/4 cup hummus
  - 2 tablespoons lemon juice
  - Salt and pepper to taste

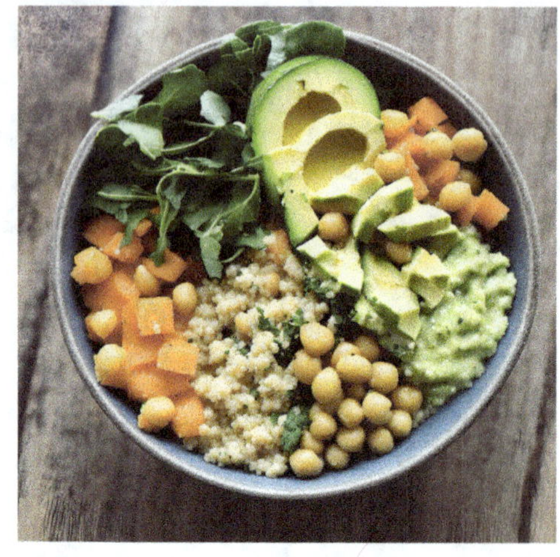

Procedure:
  1. Divide cooked quinoa, sliced avocado, cooked chickpeas, mixed greens, grated carrot, and sliced cucumber between two bowls.
  2. Drizzle lemon juice over the bowls and season with salt and pepper.
  3. Serve with a dollop of hummus on the side.

Nutritional values (per serving):
  - Calories: 450
  - Protein: 15g
  - Fat: 20g
  - Carbohydrates: 55g
  - Fiber: 15g

Shopping list:
  - Quinoa
  - Avocado
  - Chickpeas
  - Mixed greens
  - Carrot
  - Cucumber
  - Hummus
  - Lemon

62. Veggie Sushi Bowl with Brown Rice

- Preparation time: 20 minutes
- Cooking time: 30 minutes
- Portions: 2 servings

Ingredients and quantity:
  - 1 cup cooked brown rice
  - 1/2 cucumber, thinly sliced
  - 1 carrot, julienned
  - 1/2 avocado, sliced
  - 1/4 cup pickled ginger
  - 2 tablespoons rice vinegar
  - 2 tablespoons soy sauce
  - 1 tablespoon sesame oil
  - 1 tablespoon sesame seeds

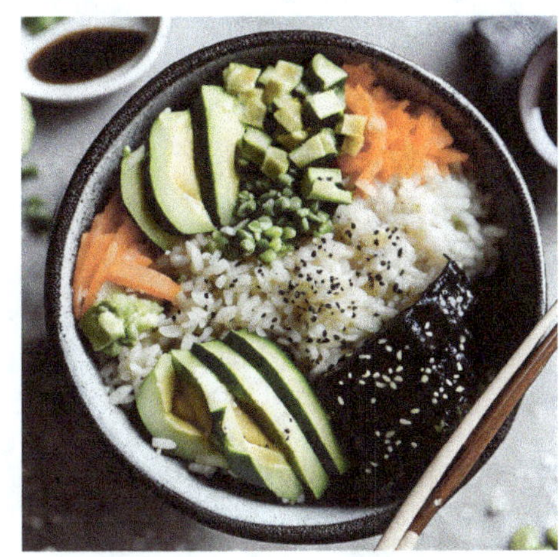

Procedure:
  1. In a small bowl, mix rice vinegar, soy sauce, and sesame oil to make the dressing.
  2. Divide cooked brown rice between two bowls.
  3. Arrange cucumber slices, julienned carrot, sliced avocado, and pickled ginger on top of the rice.
  4. Drizzle the dressing over the bowls and sprinkle with sesame seeds.

Nutritional values (per serving):
- Calories: 350
- Protein: 8g
- Fat: 10g
- Carbohydrates: 60g
- Fiber: 10g

Shopping list:
- Brown rice
- Cucumber
- Carrot
- Avocado
- Pickled ginger
- Rice vinegar
- Soy sauce
- Sesame oil
- Sesame seeds

63. Mediterranean Farro Salad

- Preparation time: 15 minutes
- Cooking time: 25 minutes
- Portions: 4 servings

Ingredients and quantity:
  - 1 cup uncooked farro
  - 1 cup cherry tomatoes, halved
  - 1/2 cup cucumber, diced
  - 1/4 cup Kalamata olives, pitted and sliced
  - 1/4 cup crumbled feta cheese (optional)
  - 2 tablespoons chopped fresh parsley
  - 2 tablespoons extra virgin olive oil
  - 1 tablespoon lemon juice
  - Salt and pepper to taste

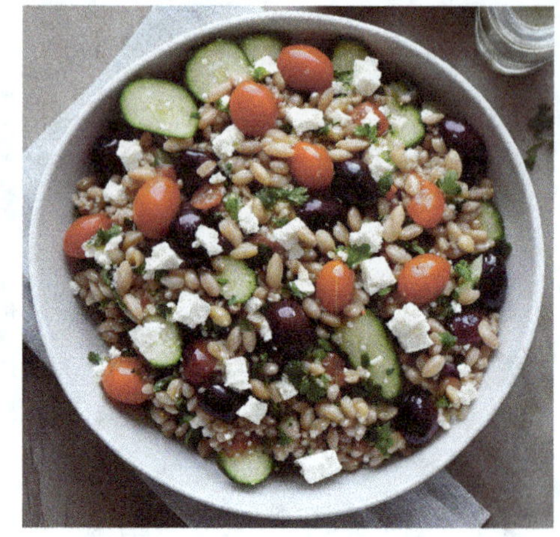

Procedure:
1. Cook farro according to package instructions until
tender. Drain and let cool.
2. In a large bowl, combine cooked farro, cherry tomatoes, cucumber, Kalamata olives,
   and crumbled feta cheese.
3. In a small bowl, whisk together extra virgin olive oil, lemon juice, salt, and pepper
   to make the dressing.
4. Pour the dressing over the salad and toss to combine.
5. Garnish with chopped fresh parsley before serving.

Nutritional values (per serving):
  - Calories: 250
  - Protein: 6g
  - Fat: 10g
  - Carbohydrates: 35g
  - Fiber: 8g

Shopping list:
 - Farro
 - Cherry tomatoes
 - Cucumber
 - Kalamata olives
 - Feta cheese (optional)
 - Fresh parsley
 - Extra virgin olive oil
 - Lemon

64. Sweet Potato and Black Bean Buddha Bowl

- Preparation time: 15 minutes
- Cooking time: 25 minutes
- Portions: 2 servings

Ingredients and quantity:
 - 1 large sweet potato, peeled and cubed
 - 1 cup cooked black beans
 - 2 cups mixed greens
 - 1 avocado, sliced
 - 1/4 cup corn kernels
 - 1/4 cup diced red bell pepper
 - 1/4 cup diced red onion
 - 2 tablespoons chopped fresh cilantro
 - 1 tablespoon olive oil
 - 1 teaspoon chili powder
 - 1/2 teaspoon cumin
 - Salt and pepper to taste

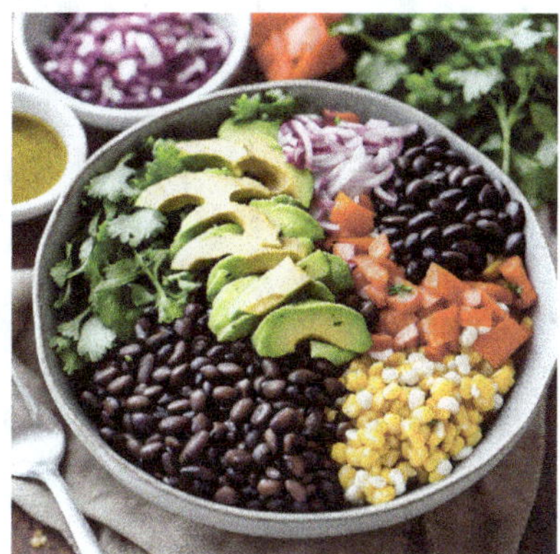

Procedure:
1. Preheat the oven to 400°F (200°C).
2. Toss sweet potato cubes with olive oil, chili powder, cumin, salt, and pepper.
3. Spread the seasoned sweet potatoes on a baking sheet and roast for 20-25 minutes until tender and lightly browned.
4. Divide mixed greens between two bowls. Top with roasted sweet potatoes, cooked black beans, avocado slices, corn kernels, diced red bell pepper, diced red onion, and chopped fresh cilantro.
5. Serve with your favorite dressing or salsa.

Nutritional values (per serving):
 - Calories: 400
 - Protein: 10g
 - Fat: 15g
 - Carbohydrates: 60g
 - Fiber: 15g

Shopping list:
 - Sweet potato
 - Black beans
 - Mixed greens
 - Avocado
 - Corn kernels
 - Red bell pepper
 - Red onion
 - Fresh cilantro
 - Olive oil
 - Chili powder
 - Cumin

65. Greek Couscous Salad with Tofu Feta

- Preparation time: 15 minutes
- Cooking time: 10 minutes
- Portions: 4 servings

Ingredients and quantity:
  - 1 cup couscous
  - 1 1/4 cups vegetable broth
  - 1 cup cherry tomatoes, halved
  - 1/2 cup diced cucumber
  - 1/4 cup Kalamata olives, pitted and sliced
  - 1/4 cup crumbled tofu feta cheese
  - 2 tablespoons chopped fresh parsley
  - 2 tablespoons extra virgin olive oil
  - 1 tablespoon lemon juice
  - Salt and pepper to taste

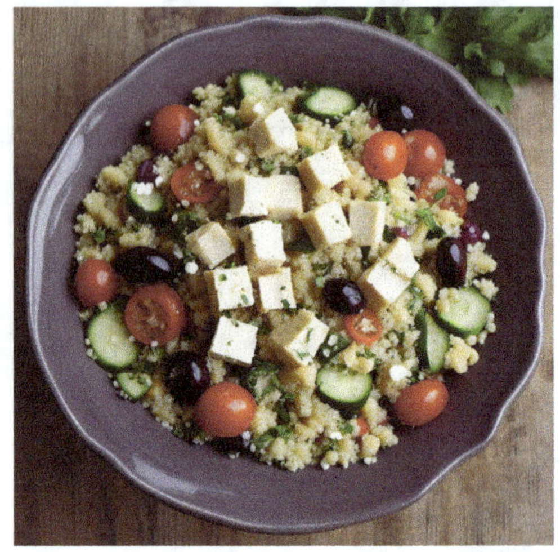

Procedure:
  1. In a saucepan, bring vegetable broth to a
     boil. Stir in couscous, cover, and remove from heat. Let it sit for 5 minutes, then fluff with a
     fork.
  2. In a large bowl, combine cooked couscous, cherry tomatoes, diced cucumber, Kalamata olives,
     crumbled tofu feta cheese, and chopped fresh parsley.
  3. In a small bowl, whisk together extra virgin olive oil, lemon juice, salt, and pepper to make the
     dressing.
  4. Pour the dressing over the salad and toss to combine.

Nutritional values (per serving):
- Calories: 300
- Protein: 8g
- Fat: 10g
- Carbohydrates: 45g
- Fiber: 5g

Shopping list:
  - Couscous
  - Vegetable broth
  - Cherry tomatoes
  - Cucumber
  - Kalamata olives
  - Tofu
  - Fresh parsley
  - Extra virgin olive oil
  - Lemon

66. Southwest Quinoa Salad with Avocado Dressing

- Preparation time: 20 minutes
  - Cooking time: 15 minutes
  - Portions: 4 servings

Ingredients and quantity:
  - 1 cup quinoa
  - 1 1/4 cups vegetable broth
  - 1 cup black beans, cooked
  - 1 cup corn kernels, cooked
  - 1 red bell pepper, diced
  - 1/2 red onion, diced
  - 1 avocado
  - 1/4 cup chopped fresh cilantro
  - 2 tablespoons lime juice
  - 2 tablespoons olive oil
  - 1 teaspoon chili powder
  - Salt and pepper to taste

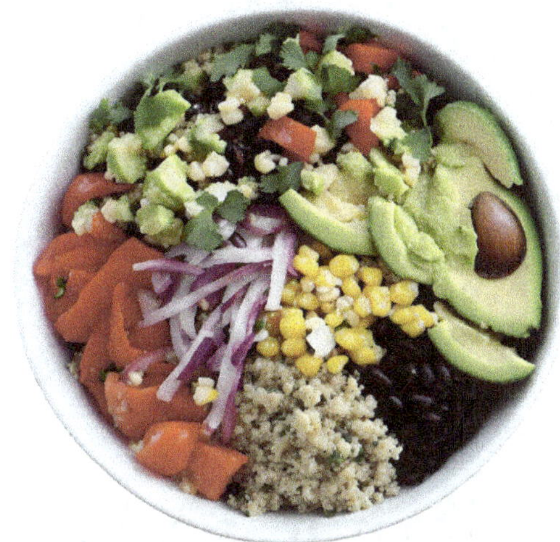

Procedure:
  1. Rinse quinoa under cold water. In a saucepan, bring vegetable broth to a boil. Add quinoa, cover, and simmer for 15 minutes or until water is absorbed. Remove from heat and let it cool.
  2. In a large bowl, combine cooked quinoa, black beans, corn kernels, diced red bell pepper, and diced red onion.
  3. In a blender, combine avocado, chopped fresh cilantro, lime juice, olive oil, chili powder, salt, and pepper. Blend until smooth and creamy to make the avocado dressing.
  4. Pour the avocado dressing over the quinoa salad and toss until well coated.

Nutritional values (per serving):
  - Calories: 350
  - Protein: 10g
  - Fat: 15g
  - Carbohydrates: 45g
  - Fiber: 10g

Shopping list:
  - Quinoa
  - Vegetable broth
  - Black beans
  - Corn kernels
  - Red bell pepper
  - Red onion
  - Avocado
  - Fresh cilantro
  - Lime
  - Olive oil
  - Chili powder

67. Asian Noodle Bowl with Tofu and Veggies

- Preparation time: 15 minutes
- Cooking time: 15 minutes
- Portions: 2 servings

Ingredients and quantity:
- 6 oz (170g) rice noodles
- 1 tablespoon sesame oil
- 8 oz (225g) firm tofu, pressed and cubed
- 2 cups mixed vegetables
  (such as bell peppers, broccoli, carrots), sliced
- 2 cloves garlic, minced
- 2 tablespoons soy sauce
- 1 tablespoon rice vinegar
- 1 tablespoon maple syrup or honey
- 1 teaspoon grated ginger
- Sesame seeds and chopped green onions for garnish

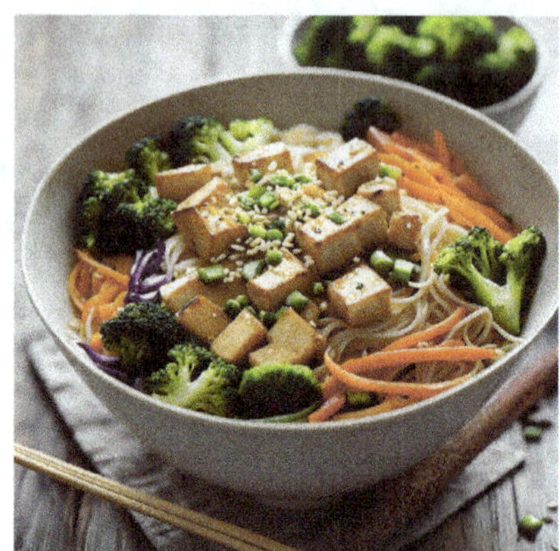

Procedure:
1. Cook rice noodles according to package instructions. Drain and set aside.
2. In a large skillet, heat sesame oil over medium heat. Add cubed tofu and cook until golden brown on all sides. Remove tofu from the skillet and set aside.
3. In the same skillet, add mixed vegetables and minced garlic. Stir-fry until vegetables are tender-crisp.
4. In a small bowl, whisk together soy sauce, rice vinegar, maple syrup or honey, and grated ginger.
5. Return tofu to the skillet. Add cooked rice noodles and the sauce mixture. Toss everything together until well combined and heated through.
6. Serve the noodle mixture in bowls, garnished with sesame seeds and chopped green onions.

Nutritional values (per serving):
- Calories: 400
- Protein: 15g
- Fat: 10g
- Carbohydrates: 65g
- Fiber: 6g

Shopping list:
- Rice noodles
- Sesame oil

- Firm tofu
- Mixed vegetables
  (bell peppers, broccoli, carrots)
- Garlic
- Soy sauce
- Rice vinegar
- Maple syrup or honey
- Ginger
- Sesame seeds
- Green onions

68. Rainbow Veggie Bowl with Turmeric Tahini Dressing

- Preparation time: 20 minutes
- Cooking time: N/A
- Portions: 2 servings

Ingredients and quantity:
  - 2 cups cooked quinoa
  - 1 cup cherry tomatoes, halved
  - 1/2 cup shredded carrots
  - 1/2 cup thinly sliced red cabbage
  - 1/2 cup sliced cucumber
  - 1/4 cup diced red bell pepper
  - 1/4 cup shelled edamame
  - 2 tablespoons chopped fresh cilantro
  - 2 tablespoons tahini
  - 1 tablespoon lemon juice
  - 1 teaspoon turmeric powder
  - 1 teaspoon maple syrup or honey
  - Salt and pepper to taste

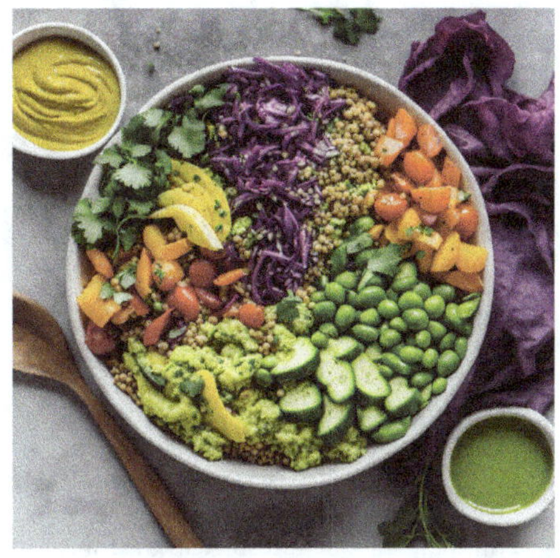

Procedure:
1. Divide cooked quinoa between two bowls.
2. Arrange cherry tomatoes, shredded carrots, sliced red cabbage, sliced cucumber, diced red bell pepper, shelled edamame, and chopped fresh cilantro on top of the quinoa.
3. In a small bowl, whisk together tahini, lemon juice, turmeric powder, maple syrup or honey, salt, and pepper to make the dressing.
4. Drizzle the turmeric tahini dressing over the veggie bowls.

Nutritional values (per serving):
  - Calories: 350
  - Protein: 12g
  - Fat: 10g
  - Carbohydrates: 55g
  - Fiber: 10g

Shopping list:
  - Quinoa
  - Cherry tomatoes
  - Carrots
  - Red cabbage
  - Cucumber
  - Red bell pepper
  - Edamame
  - Fresh cilantro
  - Tahini
  - Lemon
  - Turmeric powder
  - Maple syrup or honey

69. Caprese Quinoa Bowl with Balsamic Glaze

- Preparation time: 15 minutes
- Cooking time: 15 minutes
- Portions: 2 servings

Ingredients and quantity:
  - 1 cup cooked quinoa
  - 1 cup cherry tomatoes, halved
  - 1 cup fresh mozzarella balls
  - 1/4 cup chopped fresh basil
  - 2 tablespoons balsamic glaze
  - Salt and pepper to taste

Procedure:
  1. Divide cooked quinoa between
     two bowls.
  2. Arrange cherry tomatoes and fresh
     mozzarella balls on top of the quinoa.
  3. Sprinkle chopped fresh basil over the bowls.
  4. Drizzle balsamic glaze over the bowls.
  5. Season with salt and pepper to taste.

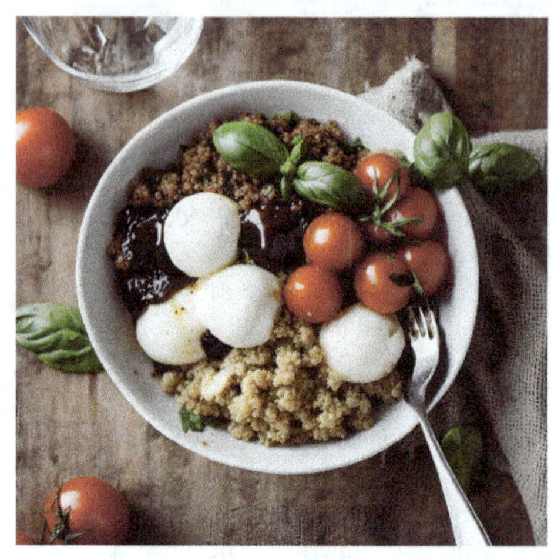

Nutritional values (per serving):
  - Calories: 300
  - Protein: 15g
  - Fat: 10g
  - Carbohydrates: 35g
  - Fiber: 5g

Shopping list:
  - Quinoa
  - Cherry tomatoes
  - Fresh mozzarella balls
  - Fresh basil
  - Balsamic glaze

70. Falafel Bowl with Hummus and Tahini Sauce

- Preparation time: 30 minutes
- Cooking time: 20 minutes
- Portions: 4 servings

Ingredients and quantity:
- 1 cup dried chickpeas, soaked overnight
- 1/2 cup chopped fresh parsley
- 1/2 cup chopped fresh cilantro
- 1 small onion, chopped
- 3 cloves garlic, minced
- 1 teaspoon ground cumin
- 1 teaspoon ground coriander
- 1/2 teaspoon baking soda
- Salt and pepper to taste
- 2 tablespoons olive oil
- 4 cups cooked quinoa
- 2 cups shredded lettuce
- 1 cucumber, diced
- 1 cup cherry tomatoes, halved
- 1/2 cup sliced red onion
- 1/4 cup chopped fresh mint
- Hummus and tahini sauce for serving

Procedure:
1. Drain and rinse the soaked chickpeas. In a food processor, combine chickpeas, parsley, cilantro, onion, garlic, cumin, coriander, baking soda, salt, and pepper. Pulse until the mixture is finely chopped and holds together when pressed.
2. Heat olive oil in a skillet over medium heat. Form the chickpea mixture into small patties and fry until golden brown on both sides, about 4 minutes per side. Remove from the skillet and drain on paper towels.
3. Assemble the falafel bowls by dividing cooked quinoa between four bowls. Top with shredded lettuce, diced cucumber, halved cherry tomatoes, sliced red onion, and chopped fresh mint.
4. Add falafel patties to each bowl and serve with hummus and tahini sauce on the side.

Nutritional values (per serving):
- Calories: 450
- Protein: 18g
- Fat: 12g
- Carbohydrates: 70g
- Fiber: 12g

Shopping list:
- Dried chickpeas
- Fresh parsley
- Fresh cilantro
- Onion
- Garlic
- Ground cumin

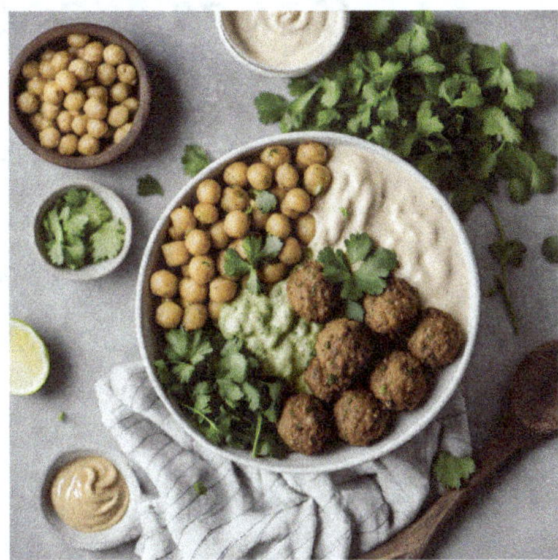

- Ground coriander
- Baking soda
- Olive oil
- Quinoa
- Lettuce
- Cucumber
- Cherry tomatoes
- Red onion
- Fresh mint
- Hummus
- Tahini sauce

Chapter 8

Baked Goods and Desserts

71. Vegan Chocolate Chip Cookies

- Preparation time: 15 minutes
- Cooking time: 10 minutes
- Portions: Makes about 24 cookies

Ingredients and quantity:
- 1/2 cup vegan butter, softened
- 1/2 cup brown sugar
- 1/4 cup granulated sugar
- 1 teaspoon vanilla extract
- 1 1/2 cups all-purpose flour
- 1/2 teaspoon baking soda
- 1/4 teaspoon salt
- 1/2 cup dairy-free chocolate chips

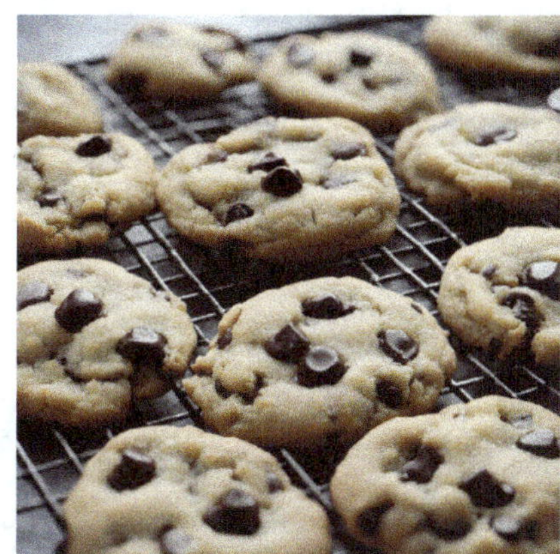

Procedure:
1. Preheat the oven to 350°F (175°C). Line a baking sheet with parchment paper.
2. In a large mixing bowl, cream together the softened vegan butter, brown sugar, granulated sugar, and vanilla extract until smooth.
3. In a separate bowl, whisk together the all-purpose flour, baking soda, and salt.
4. Gradually add the dry ingredients to the wet ingredients, mixing until well combined.
5. Fold in the dairy-free chocolate chips.
6. Drop tablespoon-sized portions of dough onto the prepared baking sheet, spacing them about 2 inches apart.
7. Bake in the preheated oven for 8-10 minutes, or until the edges are golden brown.
8. Allow the cookies to cool on the baking sheet for 5 minutes before transferring them to a wire rack to cool completely.

Nutritional values (per cookie):
- Calories: 90
- Protein: 1g
- Fat: 5g
- Carbohydrates: 11g
- Fiber: 0.5g

Shopping list:
- Vegan butter
- Brown sugar
- Granulated sugar
- Vanilla extract
- All-purpose flour
- Baking soda
- Salt
- Dairy-free chocolate chips

72. Banana Bread Muffins with Walnuts

- Preparation time: 15 minutes
- Cooking time: 20 minutes
- Portions: Makes 12 muffins

Ingredients and quantity:
- 2 ripe bananas, mashed
- 1/3 cup melted coconut oil
- 1/2 cup maple syrup
- 1/4 cup unsweetened almond milk
- 1 teaspoon vanilla extract
- 1 3/4 cups whole wheat flour
- 1 teaspoon baking soda
- 1/2 teaspoon ground cinnamon
- 1/4 teaspoon salt
- 1/2 cup chopped walnuts

Procedure:
1. Preheat the oven to 350°F (175°C). Line a muffin tin with paper liners or grease with coconut oil.
2. In a large mixing bowl, combine the mashed bananas, melted coconut oil, maple syrup, almond milk, and vanilla extract.
3. In a separate bowl, whisk together the whole wheat flour, baking soda, cinnamon, and salt.
4. Gradually add the dry ingredients to the wet ingredients, mixing until just combined.
5. Fold in the chopped walnuts.
6. Divide the batter evenly among the prepared muffin cups, filling each about 3/4 full.
7. Bake in the preheated oven for 18-20 minutes, or until a toothpick inserted into the center comes out clean.
8. Allow the muffins to cool in the tin for 5 minutes before transferring them to a wire rack to cool completely.

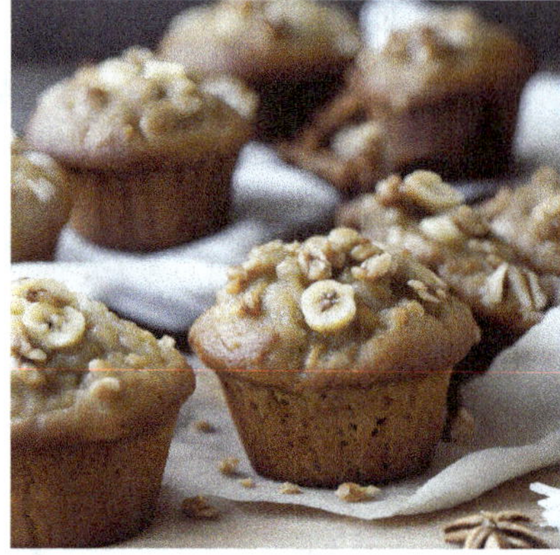

Nutritional values (per muffin):
- Calories: 180
- Protein: 3g
- Fat: 8g
- Carbohydrates: 26g
- Fiber: 3g

Shopping list:
- Ripe bananas
- Coconut oil
- Maple syrup
- Unsweetened almond milk
- Vanilla extract
- Whole wheat flour
- Baking soda
- Ground cinnamon
- Salt
- Walnut

73. Apple Cinnamon Oatmeal Cookies

- Preparation time: 20 minutes
- Cooking time: 12 minutes
- Portions: Makes about 18 cookies

Ingredients and quantity:
- 1 cup rolled oats
- 1 cup whole wheat flour
- 1 teaspoon ground cinnamon
- 1/2 teaspoon baking soda
- 1/4 teaspoon salt
- 1/4 cup coconut oil, melted
- 1/4 cup maple syrup
- 1/4 cup unsweetened applesauce
- 1 teaspoon vanilla extract
- 1/2 cup finely chopped apple

Procedure:
1. Preheat the oven to 350°F (175°C). Line a baking sheet with parchment paper.
2. In a large mixing bowl, combine the rolled oats, whole wheat flour, cinnamon, baking soda, and salt.
3. In a separate bowl, whisk together the melted coconut oil, maple syrup, applesauce, and vanilla extract.
4. Gradually add the wet ingredients to the dry ingredients, mixing until just combined.
5. Fold in the finely chopped apple.
6. Drop tablespoon-sized portions of dough onto the prepared baking sheet, spacing them about 2 inches apart.
7. Flatten each cookie slightly with the back of a spoon.
8. Bake in the preheated oven for 10-12 minutes, or until the edges are golden brown.
9. Allow the cookies to cool on the baking sheet for 5 minutes before transferring them to a wire rack to cool completely.

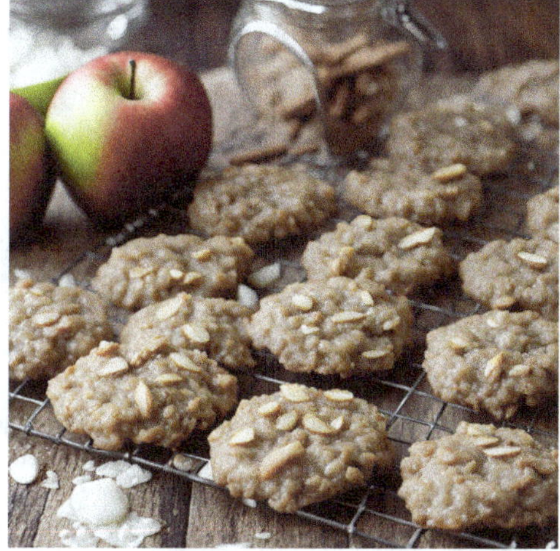

Nutritional values (per cookie):
- Calories: 90
- Protein: 1g
- Fat: 3g
- Carbohydrates: 15g
- Fiber: 1g

Shopping list:
- Rolled oats
- Whole wheat flour
- Ground cinnamon
- Baking soda
- Salt
- Coconut oil
- Maple syrup
- Unsweetened applesauce
- Vanilla extract
- Apple

74. Carrot Cake Cupcakes with Cashew Cream Frosting

- Preparation time: 25 minutes
  - Cooking time: 20 minutes
  - Portions: Makes 12 cupcakes

Ingredients and quantity:
- 1 1/2 cups grated carrots
- 1/2 cup unsweetened applesauce
- 1/4 cup melted coconut oil
- 1/3 cup maple syrup
- 1 teaspoon vanilla extract
- 1 1/4 cups whole wheat flour
- 1/2 teaspoon baking soda
- 1 teaspoon ground cinnamon
- 1/4 teaspoon ground nutmeg
- 1/4 teaspoon ground ginger
- 1/4 teaspoon salt
- 1/2 cup chopped walnuts (optional)
- 1/4 cup raisins (optional)
- For the Cashew Cream Frosting:
  - 1 cup raw cashews, soaked for at least 4 hours or overnight
  - 1/4 cup maple syrup
  - 2 tablespoons coconut oil, melted
  - 2 tablespoons lemon juice
  - 1 teaspoon vanilla extract
  - Pinch of salt

Procedure:
1. Preheat the oven to 350°F (175°C). Line a muffin tin with paper liners.
2. In a large mixing bowl, combine the grated carrots, applesauce, melted coconut oil, maple syrup, and vanilla extract.
3. In a separate bowl, whisk together the whole wheat flour, baking soda, cinnamon, nutmeg, ginger, and salt.
4. Gradually add the dry ingredients to the wet ingredients, mixing until just combined.
5. Fold in the chopped walnuts and raisins, if using.
6. Divide the batter evenly among the muffin cups, filling each about 2/3 full.
7. Bake in the preheated oven for 18-20 minutes, or until a toothpick inserted into the center comes out clean.
8. Allow the cupcakes to cool in the tin for 5 minutes before transferring them to a wire rack to cool completely.
9. While the cupcakes cool, prepare the Cashew Cream Frosting by blending all frosting ingredients in a high-speed blender until smooth and creamy.
10. Once the cupcakes are completely cooled, frost them with the Cashew Cream Frosting.

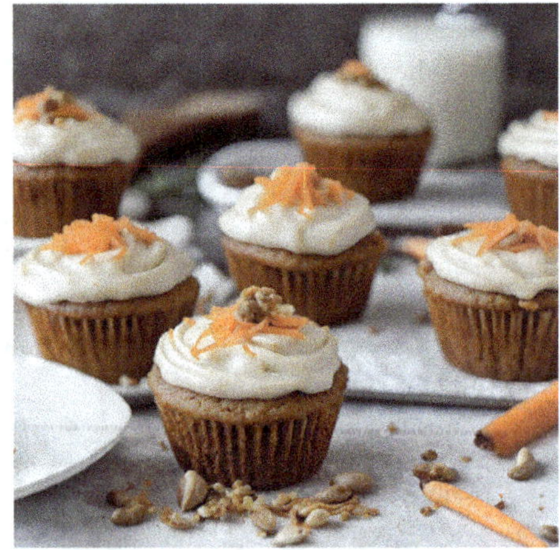

Nutritional values (per cupcake with frosting):
- Calories: 250
- Protein: 5g
- Fat: 14g
- Carbohydrates: 29g
- Fiber: 3g

Shopping list:
- Carrots
- Unsweetened applesauce
- Coconut oil
- Maple syrup
- Vanilla extract
- Whole wheat flour
- Baking soda
- Ground cinnamon
- Ground nutmeg
- Ground ginger
- Salt
- Walnuts (optional)
- Raisins (optional)
- Raw cashews
- Lemon juice

75. Blueberry Almond Flour Muffins

- Preparation time: 15 minutes
- Cooking time: 25 minutes
- Portions: Makes 12 muffins

Ingredients and quantity:
- 2 cups almond flour
- 1/4 cup coconut flour
- 1 teaspoon baking powder
- 1/4 teaspoon salt
- 1/2 cup maple syrup
- 1/4 cup almond milk
- 2 tablespoons coconut oil, melted
- 2 eggs
- 1 teaspoon vanilla extract
- 1 cup fresh or frozen blueberries

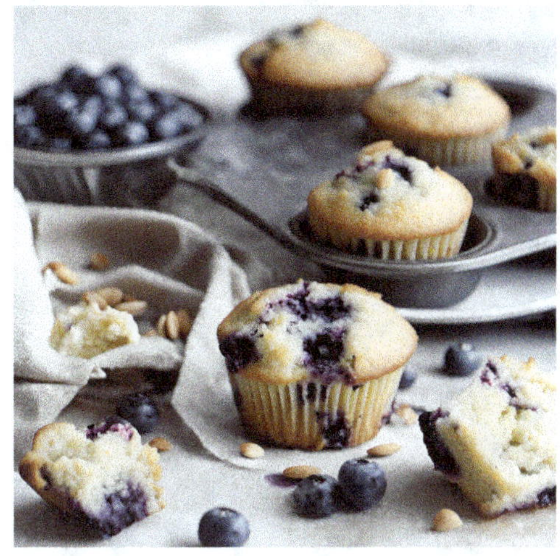

Procedure:
1. Preheat the oven to 350°F (175°C). Line a muffin tin with paper liners.
2. In a large mixing bowl, whisk together the almond flour, coconut flour, baking powder, and salt.
3. In a separate bowl, whisk together the maple syrup, almond milk, melted coconut oil, eggs, and vanilla extract.
4. Gradually add the wet ingredients to the dry ingredients, mixing until just combined.
5. Gently fold in the blueberries.
6. Divide the batter evenly among the muffin cups, filling each about 3/4 full.
7. Bake in the preheated oven for 20-25 minutes, or until a toothpick inserted into the center comes out clean.
8. Allow the muffins to cool in the tin for 5 minutes before transferring them to a wire rack to cool completely.

Nutritional values (per muffin):
- Calories: 180
- Protein: 5g
- Fat: 12g
- Carbohydrates: 15g
- Fiber: 3g

Shopping list:
- Almond flour
- Coconut flour
- Baking powder
- Salt
- Maple syrup
- Almond milk
- Coconut oil
- Eggs
- Vanilla extract
- Fresh or frozen blueberries

76. Vegan Chocolate Avocado Pudding

- Preparation time: 10 minutes
- Cooking time: N/A
- Portions: Serves 4

Ingredients and quantity:
 - 2 ripe avocados
 - 1/4 cup cocoa powder
 - 1/4 cup maple syrup
 - 1 teaspoon vanilla extract
 - Pinch of salt
 - Optional toppings: fresh berries, chopped
   nuts, shredded coconut

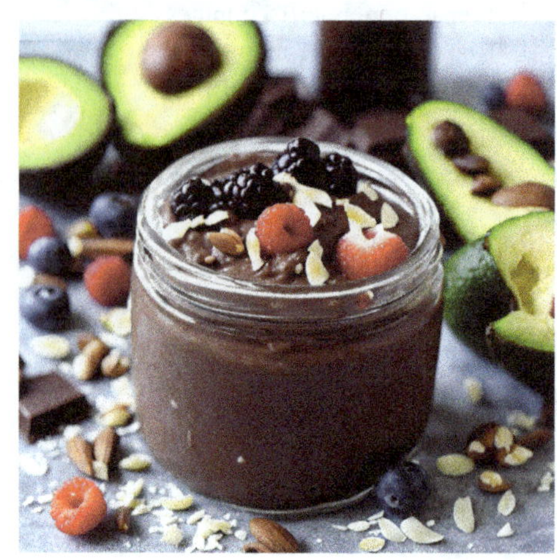

Procedure:
 1. Scoop the flesh of the avocados into a blender or
    food processor.
 2. Add the cocoa powder, maple syrup, vanilla extract, and salt.
 3. Blend until smooth and creamy, scraping down the sides as needed.
 4. Taste and adjust sweetness if necessary by adding more maple syrup.
 5. Transfer the pudding to serving bowls and refrigerate for at least 30 minutes before serving.
 6. Garnish with fresh berries, chopped nuts, or shredded coconut if desired.

Nutritional values (per serving):
 - Calories: 200
 - Protein: 3g
 - Fat: 14g
 - Carbohydrates: 22g
 - Fiber: 7g

Shopping list:
 - Ripe avocados
 - Cocoa powder
 - Maple syrup
 - Vanilla extract
 - Salt
 - Optional toppings: fresh berries,
   chopped nuts, shredded coconut

77. Pumpkin Spice Energy Balls

- Preparation time: 15 minutes
  - Cooking time: N/A
  - Portions: Makes about 12 balls

Ingredients and quantity:
  - 1 cup rolled oats
  - 1/2 cup pumpkin puree
  - 1/4 cup almond butter
  - 1/4 cup maple syrup
  - 1 teaspoon pumpkin pie spice
  - 1/4 cup shredded coconut
    (optional, for rolling)

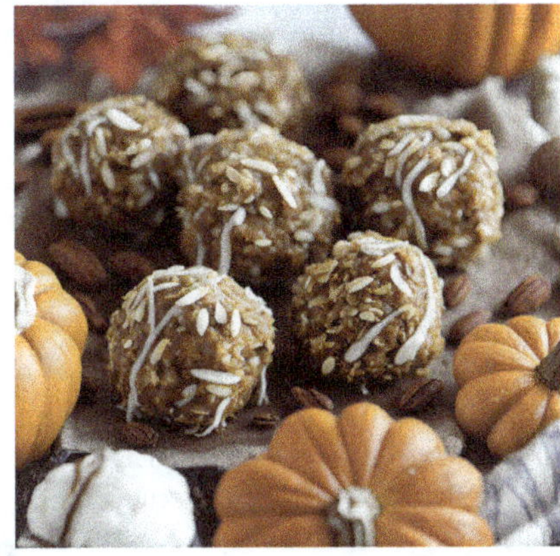

Procedure:
1. In a large mixing bowl, combine the rolled oats, pumpkin puree, almond butter, maple syrup, and pumpkin pie spice.
2. Stir until well combined and the mixture holds together.
3. Roll the mixture into tablespoon-sized balls using your hands.
4. If desired, roll the balls in shredded coconut to coat.
5. Place the energy balls on a plate or baking sheet lined with parchment paper.
6. Refrigerate for at least 30 minutes before serving.
7. Store leftovers in an airtight container in the refrigerator for up to one week.

Nutritional values (per ball):
  - Calories: 100
  - Protein: 2g
  - Fat: 4g
  - Carbohydrates: 15g
  - Fiber: 2g

Shopping list:
- Rolled oats
- Pumpkin puree
- Almond butter
- Maple syrup
- Pumpkin pie spice
- Shredded coconut (optional)

78. Raspberry Lemon Scones

- Preparation time: 15 minutes
- Cooking time: 20 minutes
- Portions: Makes 8 scones

Ingredients and quantity:
- 2 cups all-purpose flour
- 1/4 cup granulated sugar
- 1 tablespoon baking powder
- 1/2 teaspoon salt
- Zest of 1 lemon
- 1/2 cup cold unsalted butter, cubed
- 1/2 cup fresh raspberries
- 3/4 cup heavy cream, plus extra for brushing
- 1 teaspoon vanilla extract

Procedure:
1. Preheat the oven to 400°F (200°C) and line a baking sheet with parchment paper.
2. In a large bowl, whisk together the flour, sugar, baking powder, salt, and lemon zest.
3. Cut in the cold butter using a pastry cutter or your fingers until the mixture resembles coarse crumbs.
4. Gently fold in the raspberries.
5. In a separate bowl, mix together the heavy cream and vanilla extract.
6. Slowly add the cream mixture to the dry ingredients, stirring until just combined.
7. Turn the dough out onto a lightly floured surface and gently knead it a few times until it comes together.
8. Pat the dough into a circle about 1 inch thick. Cut the circle into 8 wedges.
9. Place the scones on the prepared baking sheet and brush the tops with a little extra cream.
10. Bake for 18-20 minutes, or until the scones are golden brown and cooked through.
11. Allow the scones to cool slightly before serving.

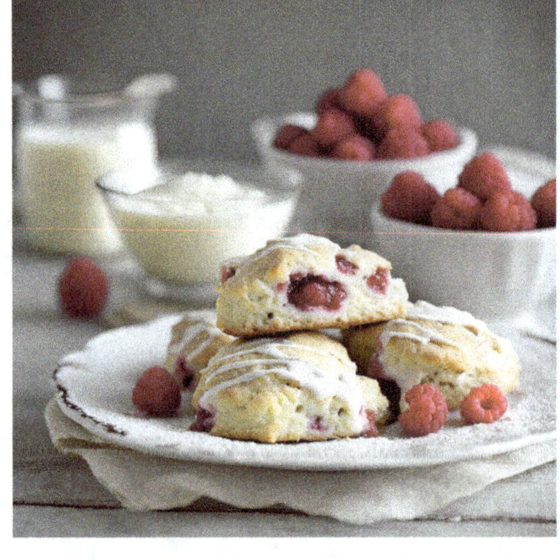

Nutritional values (per scone):
- Calories: 270
- Protein: 3g
- Fat: 15g
- Carbohydrates: 31g
- Fiber: 1g

Shopping list:
- All-purpose flour
- Granulated sugar
- Baking powder
- Salt
- Lemon
- Unsalted butter
- Fresh raspberries
- Heavy cream
- Vanilla extract

79. Coconut Flour Banana Bread

- Preparation time: 15 minutes
- Cooking time: 45-50 minutes
- Portions: Makes 1 loaf (10 slices)

Ingredients and quantity:
- 3 ripe bananas, mashed
- 3 eggs
- 1/4 cup coconut oil, melted
- 1/4 cup maple syrup
- 1 teaspoon vanilla extract
- 1/2 cup coconut flour
- 1 teaspoon baking soda
- 1/2 teaspoon ground cinnamon
- Pinch of salt
- Optional add-ins: chopped nuts, chocolate chips

Procedure:
1. Preheat the oven to 350°F (175°C). Grease a 9x5-inch loaf pan and set aside.
2. In a large mixing bowl, combine the mashed bananas, eggs, melted coconut oil, maple syrup, and vanilla extract.
3. In a separate bowl, whisk together the coconut flour, baking soda, cinnamon, and salt.
4. Gradually add the dry ingredients to the wet ingredients, stirring until well combined.
5. If using, fold in the optional add-ins such as chopped nuts or chocolate chips.
6. Pour the batter into the prepared loaf pan and smooth the top with a spatula.
7. Bake for 45-50 minutes, or until a toothpick inserted into the center comes out clean.
8. Allow the banana bread to cool in the pan for 10 minutes before transferring it to a wire rack to cool completely.
9. Slice and serve.

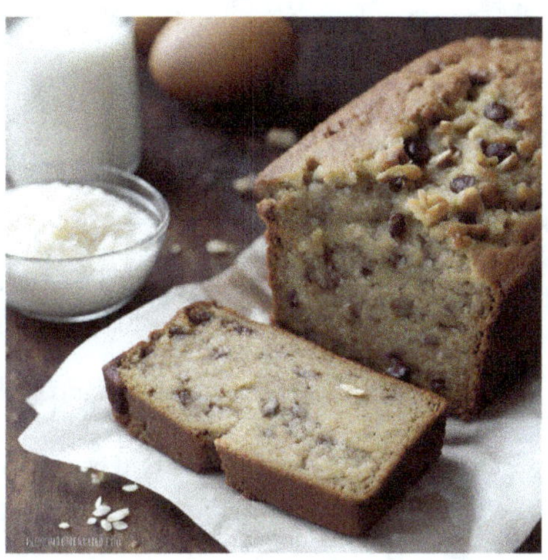

Nutritional values (per slice):
- Calories: 180
- Protein: 4g
- Fat: 9g
- Carbohydrates: 21g
- Fiber: 4g

Shopping list:
- Ripe bananas
- Eggs
- Coconut oil
- Maple syrup
- Vanilla extract
- Coconut flour
- Baking soda
- Ground cinnamon
- Salt
- Optional add-ins: chopped nuts, chocolate chips

80. Almond Butter Chocolate Chip Blondies

- Preparation time: 10 minutes
- Cooking time: 20-25 minutes
- Portions: Makes 12 blondies

Ingredients and quantity:
 - 1 cup almond butter
 - 1/2 cup maple syrup
 - 1 egg
 - 1 teaspoon vanilla extract
 - 1/2 teaspoon baking soda
 - 1/4 teaspoon salt
 - 1/2 cup dark chocolate chips
 - Optional toppings: flaky sea salt

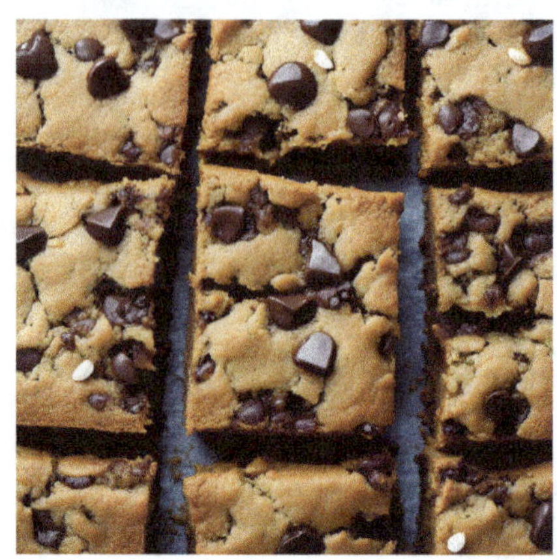

Procedure:
1. Preheat the oven to 350°F (175°C). Grease an 8x8-inch baking dish and line it with parchment paper, leaving some overhang on the sides for easy removal.
2. In a large mixing bowl, whisk together the almond butter, maple syrup, egg, and vanilla extract until smooth.
3. Add the baking soda and salt, and mix until well combined.
4. Fold in the dark chocolate chips.
5. Pour the batter into the prepared baking dish and spread it out evenly with a spatula.
6. If desired, sprinkle the top with flaky sea salt.
7. Bake for 20-25 minutes, or until the edges are golden brown and a toothpick inserted into the center comes out clean.
8. Allow the blondies to cool completely in the pan before slicing and serving.

Nutritional values (per blondie):
 - Calories: 200
 - Protein: 5g
 - Fat: 15g
 - Carbohydrates: 15g
 - Fiber: 2g

Shopping list:
 - Almond butter
 - Maple syrup
 - Egg
 - Vanilla extract
 - Baking soda
 - Salt
 - Dark chocolate chips
 - Optional: flaky sea salt

Beverages and Smoothies

81. Green Detox Smoothie

- Preparation time: 5 minutes
- Cooking time: N/A
- Portions: 1 serving

Ingredients and quantity:
- 1 cup spinach
- 1/2 cup kale
- 1/2 green apple, cored and chopped
- 1/2 cucumber, chopped
- 1/2 lemon, juiced
- 1 tablespoon fresh ginger, grated
- 1 cup coconut water
- Ice cubes (optional)

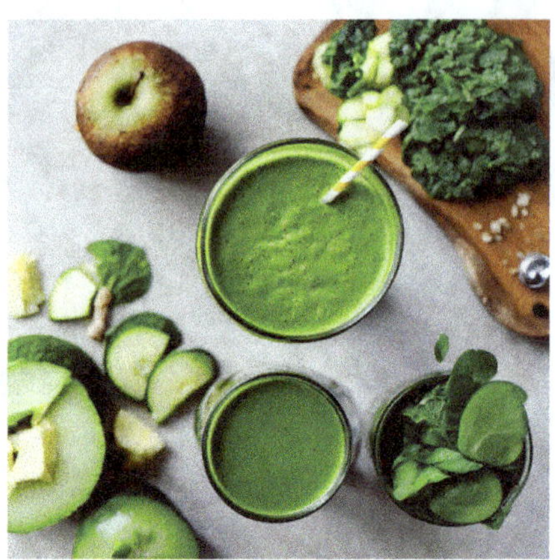

Procedure:
1. In a blender, combine the spinach, kale, green apple, cucumber, lemon juice, grated ginger, and coconut water.
2. Blend until smooth and creamy.
3. If desired, add ice cubes and blend again until smooth.
4. Pour into a glass and serve immediately.

Nutritional values (per serving):
- Calories: 90
- Protein: 3g
- Fat: 1g
- Carbohydrates: 20g
- Fiber: 6g

Shopping list:
- Spinach
- Kale
- Green apple
- Cucumber
- Lemon
- Fresh ginger
- Coconut water

82. Golden Milk Latte with Turmeric

- Preparation time: 5 minutes
- Cooking time: 5 minutes
- Portions: 1 serving

Ingredients and quantity:
- 1 cup unsweetened almond milk
- 1 teaspoon ground turmeric
- 1/2 teaspoon ground cinnamon
- 1/4 teaspoon ground ginger
- Pinch of black pepper
- 1 teaspoon honey or maple syrup (optional)
- Dash of vanilla extract

Procedure:
1. In a small saucepan, heat the almond milk over medium heat until warm but not boiling.
2. Whisk in the ground turmeric, cinnamon, ginger, black pepper, honey or maple syrup (if using), and vanilla extract.
3. Continue to heat, whisking occasionally, for about 5 minutes until the mixture is hot and well combined.
4. Pour the golden milk latte into a mug and serve warm.

Nutritional values (per serving):
- Calories: 40
- Protein: 1g
- Fat: 2g
- Carbohydrates: 6g
- Fiber: 1g

Shopping list:
- Unsweetened almond milk
- Ground turmeric
- Ground cinnamon
- Ground ginger
- Black pepper
- Honey or maple syrup
- Vanilla extract

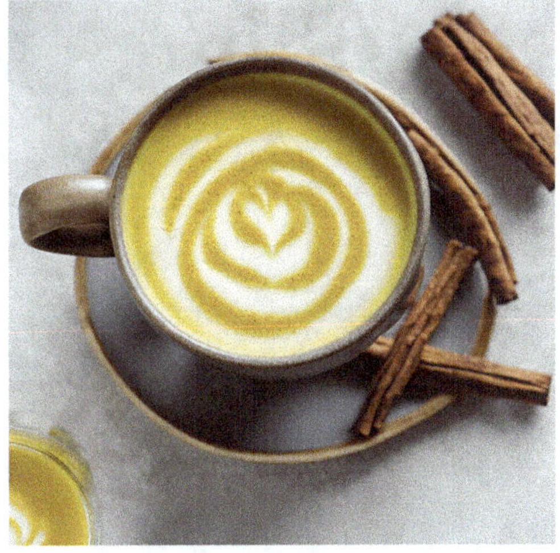

83. Berry Blast Smoothie with Spinach

- Preparation time: 5 minutes
- Cooking time: N/A
- Portions: 1 serving

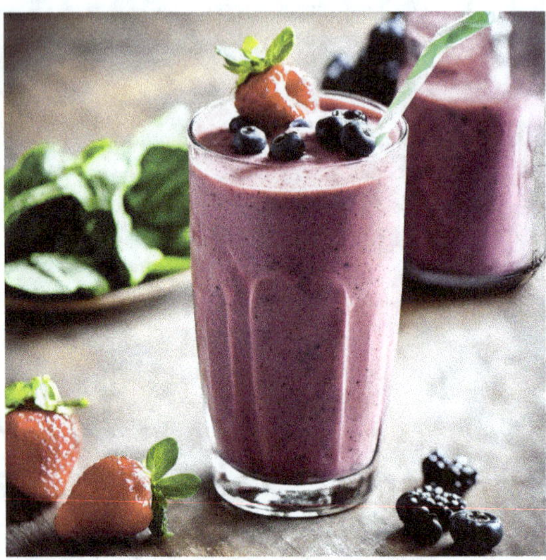

Ingredients and quantity:
- 1 cup mixed berries (strawberries, blueberries, raspberries)
- 1/2 banana
- 1 cup spinach
- 1/2 cup unsweetened almond milk
- 1 tablespoon chia seeds
- Ice cubes (optional)

Procedure:
1. In a blender, combine the mixed berries, banana, spinach, almond milk, and chia seeds.
2. Blend until smooth and creamy.
3. If desired, add ice cubes and blend again until smooth.
4. Pour into a glass and serve immediately.

Nutritional values (per serving):
- Calories: 150
- Protein: 5g
- Fat: 5g
- Carbohydrates: 25g
- Fiber: 8g

Shopping list:
- Mixed berries
  (strawberries, blueberries, raspberries)
- Banana
- Spinach
- Unsweetened almond milk
- Chia seeds

84. Iced Matcha Latte

- Preparation time: 5 minutes
- Cooking time: N/A
- Portions: 1 serving

Ingredients and quantity:
  - 1 teaspoon matcha powder
  - 1 cup unsweetened almond milk
  - 1/2 teaspoon honey or maple syrup (optional)
  - Ice cubes

Procedure:
  1. In a glass, whisk together the matcha powder and a splash of almond milk until smooth.
  2. Add the remaining almond milk and honey or maple syrup (if using), and stir until well combined.
  3. Add ice cubes to a separate glass, then pour the matcha mixture over the ice.
  4. Stir well and enjoy immediately.

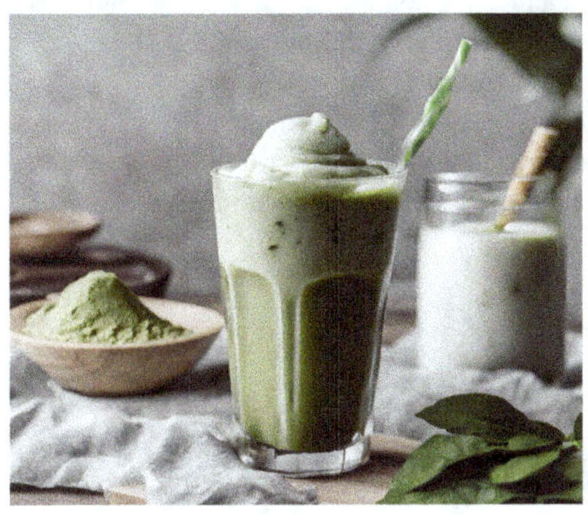

  - Fiber: 1g

Nutritional values (per serving):
  - Calories: 30
  - Protein: 1g
  - Fat: 1g
  - Carbohydrates: 4g

Shopping list:
  - Matcha powder
  - Unsweetened almond milk
  - Honey or maple syrup (optional)

85. Pineapple Mango Smoothie with Coconut Milk

- Preparation time: 5 minutes
- Cooking time: N/A
- Portions: 1 serving

Ingredients and quantity:
- 1/2 cup pineapple chunks
- 1/2 cup mango chunks
- 1/2 banana
- 1/2 cup coconut milk
- 1/2 cup water or coconut water
- Ice cubes

Procedure:
1. In a blender, combine the pineapple chunks, mango chunks, banana, coconut milk, and water or coconut water.
2. Blend until smooth and creamy.
3. If desired, add ice cubes and blend again until smooth.
4. Pour into a glass and serve immediately.

Nutritional values (per serving):
- Calories: 200
- Protein: 2g
- Fat: 10g
- Carbohydrates: 28g
- Fiber: 4g

Shopping list:
- Pineapple chunks
- Mango chunks
- Banana
- Coconut milk
- Water or coconut water

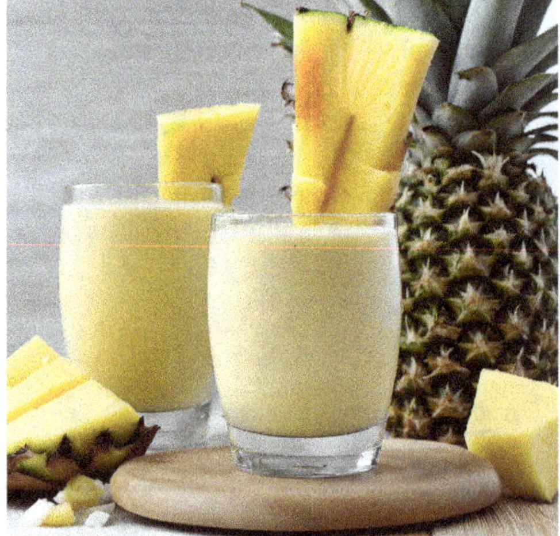

86. Beetroot and Berry Smoothie

- Preparation time: 5 minutes
- Cooking time: N/A
- Portions: 1 serving

Ingredients and quantity:
- 1/2 cup cooked beetroot, chopped
- 1/2 cup mixed berries
  (strawberries, raspberries, blueberries)
- 1/2 cup plain Greek yogurt
- 1/2 cup unsweetened almond milk
- 1 tablespoon honey or maple syrup
  (optional)
- Ice cubes

Procedure:
1. In a blender, combine the cooked beetroot, mixed berries, Greek yogurt,
   almond milk, and honey or maple syrup (if using).
2. Blend until smooth and creamy.
3. If desired, add ice cubes and blend again until smooth.
4. Pour into a glass and serve immediately.

Nutritional values (per serving):
- Calories: 150
- Protein: 10g
- Fat: 3g
- Carbohydrates: 25g
- Fiber: 5g

Shopping list:
- Cooked beetroot
- Mixed berries
  (strawberries, raspberries, blueberries)
- Plain Greek yogurt
- Unsweetened almond milk
- Honey or maple syrup (optional)

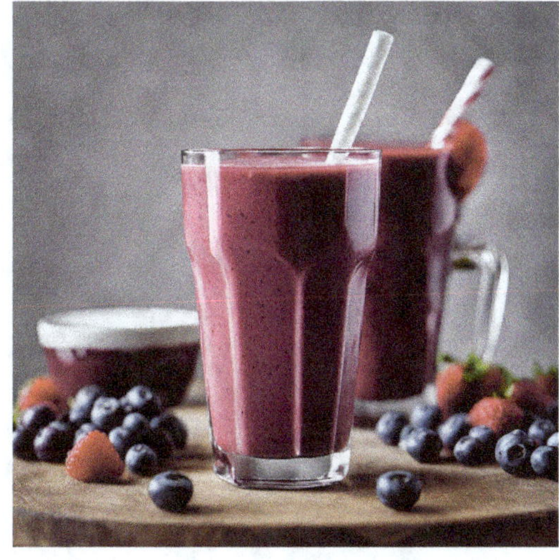

87. Cucumber Mint Lemonade

- Preparation time: 10 minutes
- Cooking time: N/A
- Portions: 2 servings

Ingredients and quantity:
- 1 cucumber, peeled and chopped
- Handful of fresh mint leaves
- 1/4 cup fresh lemon juice
- 2 tablespoons honey or agave syrup
- 2 cups cold water
- Ice cubes

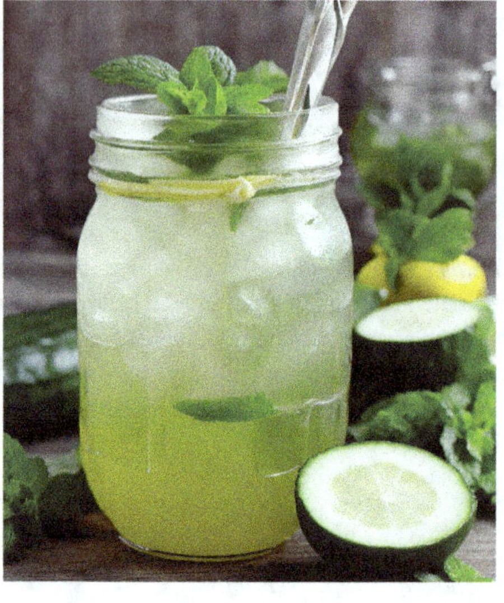

Procedure:
1. In a blender, combine the chopped cucumber, fresh mint leaves, lemon juice, honey or agave syrup, and cold water.
2. Blend until smooth.
3. Strain the mixture through a fine mesh sieve into a pitcher to remove any pulp.
4. Serve over ice cubes in glasses, garnished with cucumber slices and mint leaves if desired.

Nutritional values (per serving):
- Calories: 45
- Protein: 1g
- Fat: 0g
- Carbohydrates: 12g
- Fiber: 1g

Shopping list:
- Cucumber
- Fresh mint leaves
- Lemon
- Honey or agave syrup

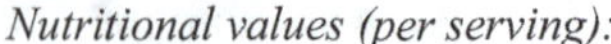

88. Vegan Pumpkin Spice Latte

- Preparation time: 10 minutes
- Cooking time: 5 minutes
- Portions: 1 serving

Ingredients and quantity:
- 1 cup unsweetened almond milk
- 2 tablespoons pumpkin puree
- 1 tablespoon maple syrup
- 1/2 teaspoon pumpkin pie spice
- 1/2 teaspoon vanilla extract
- 1/2 cup strong brewed coffee or espresso
- Vegan whipped cream (optional)
- Ground cinnamon (for garnish)

Procedure:
1. In a small saucepan, heat the almond milk, pumpkin puree, maple syrup, pumpkin pie spice, and vanilla extract over medium heat until hot but not boiling, whisking occasionally.
2. Remove from heat and froth the mixture using a frother or whisk until foamy.
3. Pour the hot coffee or espresso into a mug, then top with the pumpkin spice mixture.
4. If desired, add vegan whipped cream on top and sprinkle with ground cinnamon.

Nutritional values (per serving):
- Calories: 80
- Protein: 1g
- Fat: 2g
- Carbohydrates: 16g
- Fiber: 1g

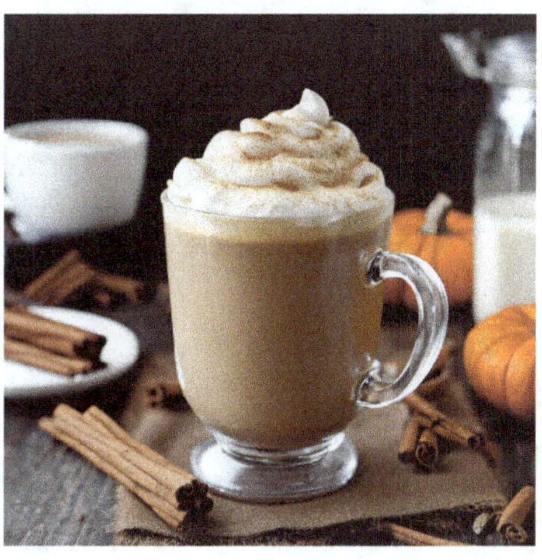

Shopping list:
- Unsweetened almond milk
- Pumpkin puree
- Maple syrup
- Pumpkin pie spice
- Vanilla extract
- Strong brewed coffee or espresso
- Vegan whipped cream
- Ground cinnamon

89. Watermelon Cucumber Cooler

- Preparation time: 10 minutes
- Cooking time: N/A
- Portions: 2 servings

Ingredients and quantity:
 - 2 cups cubed watermelon
- 1/2 cucumber, peeled and chopped
- 1 tablespoon fresh lime juice
- 1 tablespoon honey or agave syrup
- 1 cup cold water
- Ice cubes

Procedure:
1. In a blender, combine the cubed watermelon, chopped cucumber, lime juice, honey or agave syrup, and cold water.
2. Blend until smooth.
3. Strain the mixture through a fine mesh sieve into a pitcher to remove any pulp.
4. Serve over ice cubes in glasses, garnished with cucumber slices and lime wedges if desired.

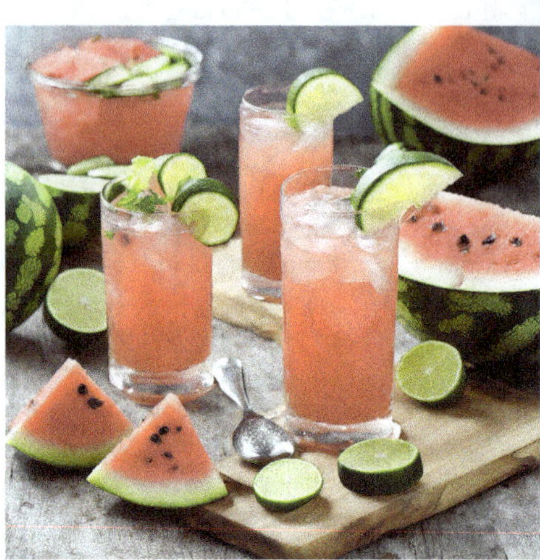

Nutritional values (per serving):
 - Calories: 70
 - Protein: 1g
 - Fat: 0g
 - Carbohydrates: 18g
 - Fiber: 1g

Shopping list:
 - Watermelon
 - Cucumber
 - Fresh lime
 - Honey or agave syrup

90. Kiwi Kale Smoothie with Ginger

- Preparation time: 5 minutes
- Cooking time: N/A
- Portions: 1 serving

Ingredients and quantity:
- 1 kiwi, peeled and chopped
- 1 cup chopped kale leaves
- 1/2 banana
- 1/2-inch piece of fresh ginger, peeled and chopped
- 1/2 cup unsweetened almond milk
- 1/2 cup plain Greek yogurt
- 1 tablespoon honey or maple syrup (optional)
- Ice cubes

Procedure:
1. In a blender, combine the chopped kiwi, kale leaves, banana, chopped ginger, almond milk, Greek yogurt, and honey or maple syrup (if using).
2. Blend until smooth and creamy.
3. If desired, add ice cubes and blend again until smooth.
4. Pour into a glass and serve immediately.

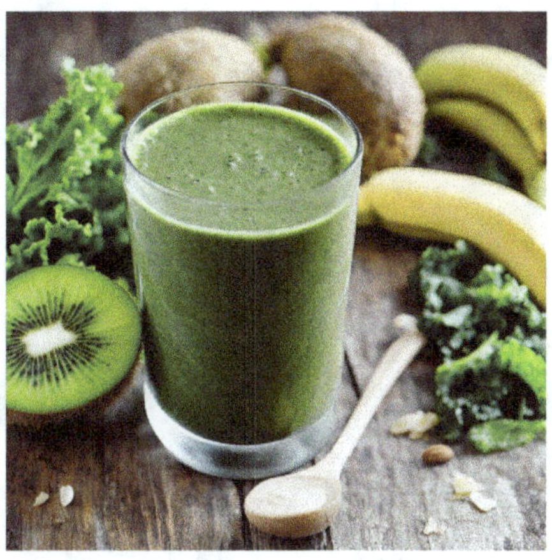

Nutritional values (per serving):
- Calories: 150
- Protein: 8g
- Fat: 3g
- Carbohydrates: 25g
- Fiber: 5g

Shopping list:
- Kiwi
- Kale leaves
- Banana
- Fresh ginger
- Unsweetened almond milk
- Plain Greek yogurt
- Honey or maple syrup (optional)

Sauces, Dressings, and Condiments

91. Classic Marinara Sauce

- Preparation time: 10 minutes
- Cooking time: 30 minutes
- Portions: Makes about 4 cups

Ingredients and quantity:
- 2 tablespoons olive oil
- 1 onion, finely chopped
- 3 cloves garlic, minced
- 1 can (28 oz) crushed tomatoes
- 1 can (14 oz) diced tomatoes
- 2 tablespoons tomato paste
- 1 teaspoon dried oregano
- 1 teaspoon dried basil
- 1/2 teaspoon dried thyme
- Salt and pepper to taste

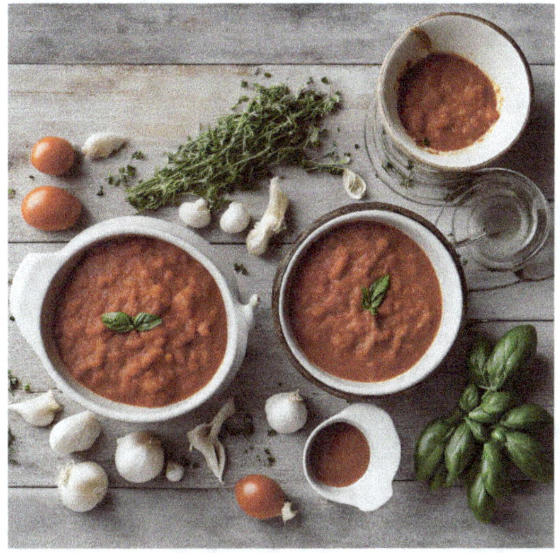

Procedure:
1. In a large saucepan, heat the olive oil over medium heat. Add the chopped onion and sauté until translucent, about 5 minutes.
2. Add the minced garlic and sauté for another 1-2 minutes until fragrant.
3. Pour in the crushed tomatoes, diced tomatoes, and tomato paste. Stir to combine.
4. Add the dried oregano, dried basil, dried thyme, salt, and pepper. Stir well.
5. Bring the sauce to a simmer, then reduce the heat to low and let it cook uncovered for about 20-25 minutes, stirring occasionally, until the sauce thickens.
6. Taste and adjust seasoning if needed.
7. Remove from heat and let the sauce cool slightly before serving or storing.

Nutritional values (per 1/2 cup serving):
- Calories: 60
- Protein: 2g
- Fat: 3g
- Carbohydrates: 9g
- Fiber: 2g

Shopping list:
- Olive oil
- Onion
- Garlic
- Crushed tomatoes
- Diced tomatoes
- Tomato paste
- Dried oregano
- Dried basil
- Dried thyme
- Salt
- Pepper

92. Vegan Cashew Cheese Sauce

- Preparation time: 10 minutes
- Cooking time: 5 minutes
- Portions: Makes about 2 cups

Ingredients and quantity:
- 1 cup raw cashews, soaked in water for 4 hours or overnight
- 1 cup unsweetened almond milk
- 1/4 cup nutritional yeast
- 2 tablespoons lemon juice
- 1 tablespoon apple cider vinegar
- 1/2 teaspoon garlic powder
- 1/2 teaspoon onion powder
- Salt and pepper to taste

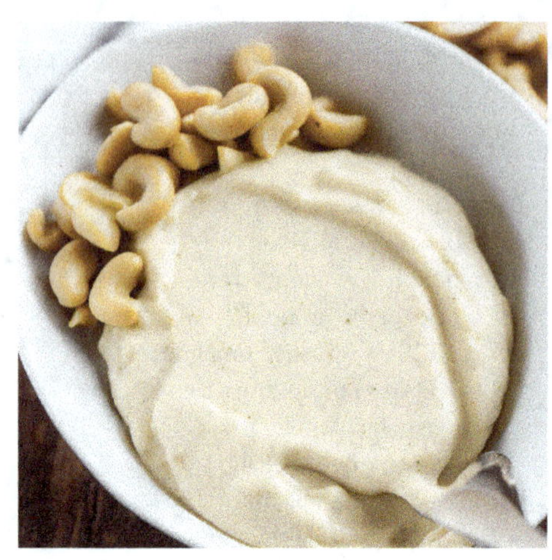

Procedure:
1. Drain and rinse the soaked cashews.
2. In a blender, combine the soaked cashews, almond milk, nutritional yeast, lemon juice, apple cider vinegar, garlic powder, onion powder, salt, and pepper.
3. Blend on high speed until smooth and creamy, scraping down the sides as needed.
4. If the sauce is too thick, add more almond milk, a tablespoon at a time, until desired consistency is reached.
5. Taste and adjust seasoning if needed.
6. Transfer the sauce to a saucepan and heat over medium-low heat, stirring constantly, until warmed through.
7. Remove from heat and serve immediately, or store in an airtight container in the refrigerator for up to 1 week.

Nutritional values (per 1/4 cup serving):
- Calories: 100
- Protein: 4g
- Fat: 7g
- Carbohydrates: 6g
- Fiber: 1g

Shopping list:
- Raw cashews
- Unsweetened almond milk
- Nutritional yeast
- Lemon
- Apple cider vinegar
- Garlic powder
- Onion powder
- Salt
- Pepper

93. Homemade Pesto with Basil and Pine Nuts

- Preparation time: 10 minutes
- Cooking time: N/A
- Portions: Makes about 1 cup

Ingredients and quantity:
  - 2 cups fresh basil leaves, packed
- 1/2 cup pine nuts
- 1/2 cup grated Parmesan cheese
  (optional for vegan version)
- 3 cloves garlic
- 1/4 cup extra-virgin olive oil
- Salt and pepper to taste

Procedure:
1. In a food processor, combine the basil leaves, pine nuts, grated Parmesan cheese (if using), and garlic cloves.
2. Pulse until coarsely chopped.
3. With the food processor running, slowly drizzle in the olive oil until the pesto reaches your desired consistency.
4. Season with salt and pepper to taste, and pulse again to combine.
5. Taste and adjust seasoning if needed.
6. Transfer the pesto to a jar or airtight container and store in the refrigerator for up to 1 week.

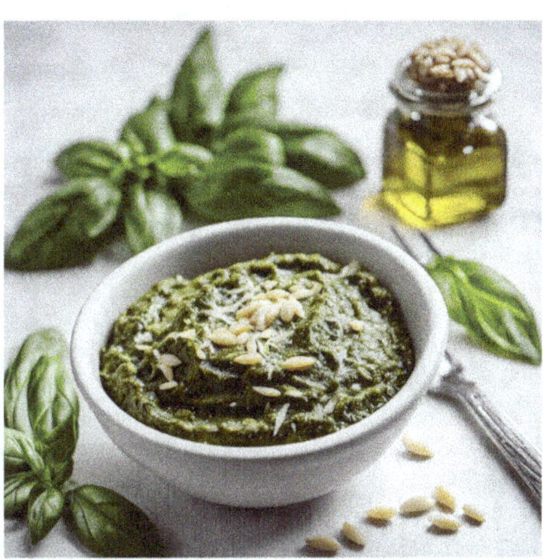

Nutritional values (per tablespoon serving):
  - Calories: 80
  - Protein: 2g
  - Fat: 8g
  - Carbohydrates: 1g
  - Fiber: 0g

Shopping list:
  - Fresh basil leaves
  - Pine nuts
  - Parmesan cheese (optional)
  - Garlic
  - Extra-virgin olive oil
  - Salt
  - Pepper

94. Balsamic Vinaigrette Dressing

- Preparation time: 5 minutes
- Cooking time: N/A
- Portions:Makes about 1/2 cup

Ingredients and quantity:
  - 1/4 cup balsamic vinegar
  - 1/4 cup extra-virgin olive oil
  - 1 tablespoon Dijon mustard
  - 1 teaspoon honey or maple syrup
    (optional for vegan version)
  - 1 clove garlic, minced
  - Salt and pepper to taste

Procedure:
  1. In a small bowl, whisk together the balsamic
     vinegar, extra-virgin olive oil, Dijon mustard,
     honey or maple syrup (if using), and minced
     garlic until well combined.
  2. Season with salt and pepper to taste, and whisk
     again until emulsified.
  3. Taste and adjust seasoning if needed.
  4. Use immediately as a dressing for salads, or
     store in an airtight container in the refrigerator
     for up to 1 week.

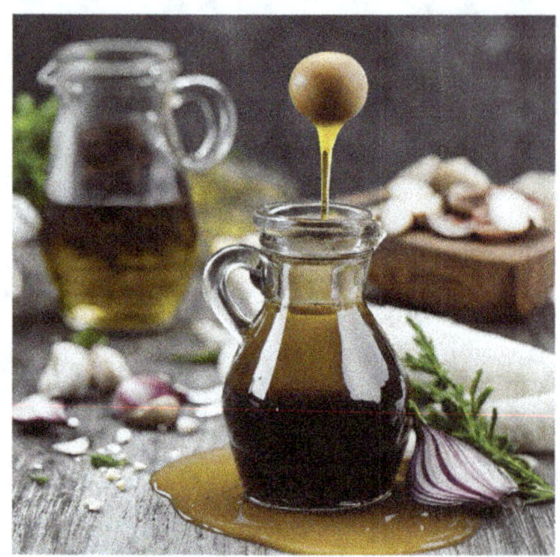

Nutritional values (per tablespoon serving):
  - Calories: 70
  - Protein: 0g
  - Fat: 7g
  - Carbohydrates: 2g
  - Fiber: 0g

Shopping list:
  - Balsamic vinegar
  - Extra-virgin olive oil
  - Dijon mustard
  - Honey or maple syrup (optional)
  - Garlic
  - Salt
  - Pepper

95. Tahini Garlic Sauce

- Preparation time: 5 minutes
- Cooking time: N/A
- Portions: Makes about 1/2 cup

Ingredients and quantity:
- 1/4 cup tahini
- 2 tablespoons lemon juice
- 1 clove garlic, minced
- 2-3 tablespoons water
- Salt to taste

Procedure:
1. In a small bowl, whisk together the tahini, lemon juice, minced garlic, and 2 tablespoons of water until smooth.
2. If the sauce is too thick, add an additional tablespoon of water and whisk again until desired consistency is reached.
3. Season with salt to taste, and whisk until well combined.
4. Taste and adjust seasoning if needed.
5. Use immediately as a sauce for salads, roasted vegetables, or grain bowls, or store in an airtight container in the refrigerator for up to 1 week.

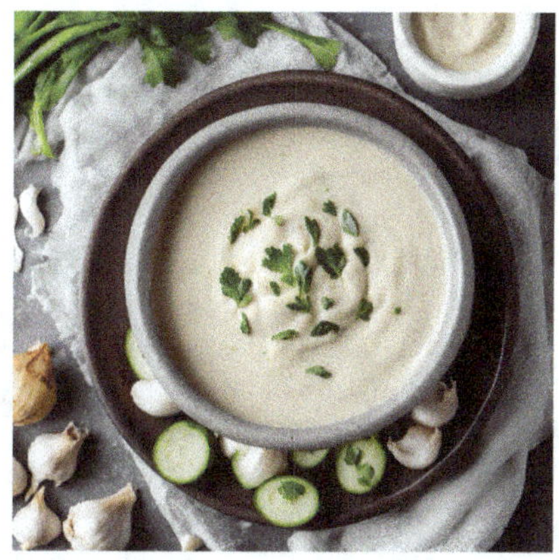

Nutritional values (per tablespoon serving):
- Calories: 60
- Protein: 2g
- Fat: 5g
- Carbohydrates: 3g
- Fiber: 1g

Shopping list:
- Tahini
- Lemon
- Garlic
- Salt

96 Vegan Ranch Dressing

- Preparation time: 10 minutes
- Cooking time: N/A
- Portions: Makes about 1 cup

Ingredients and quantity:
  - 1/2 cup vegan mayonnaise
  - 1/4 cup unsweetened almond milk (or any non-dairy milk)

- 1 tablespoon lemon juice
- 1 clove garlic, minced
- 1 teaspoon onion powder
- 1 teaspoon dried parsley
- 1/2 teaspoon dried dill
- Salt and pepper to taste

Procedure:
  1. In a small bowl, whisk together the vegan mayonnaise, unsweetened almond milk, lemon juice, minced garlic, onion powder, dried parsley, and dried dill until smooth.
  2. Season with salt and pepper to taste, and whisk again until well combined.
  3. Taste and adjust seasoning if needed.
  4. Use immediately as a dressing for salads or veggie dip, or store in an airtight container in the refrigerator for up to 1 week.

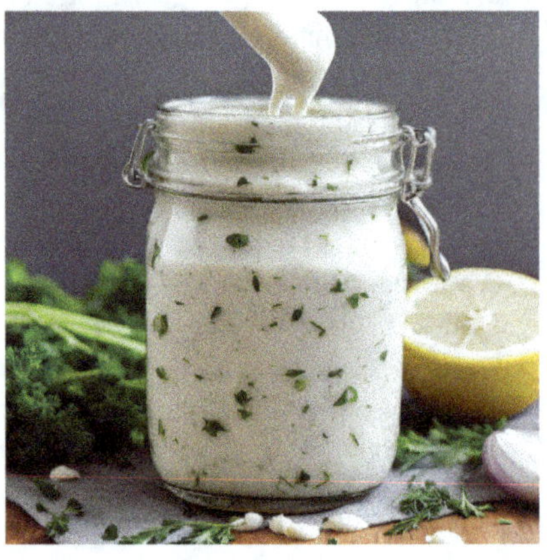

Nutritional values (per tablespoon serving):
  - Calories: 30
  - Protein: 0g
  - Fat: 3g
  - Carbohydrates: 0g
  - Fiber: 0g

Shopping list:
  - Vegan mayonnaise
  - Unsweetened almond milk
  - Lemon
  - Garlic
  - Onion powder
  - Dried parsley
  - Dried dill
  - Salt
  - Pepper

97. Chimichurri Sauce with Fresh Herbs

- Preparation time: 10 minutes
- Cooking time: N/A
- Portions: Makes about 1 cup

Ingredients and quantity:
  - 1 cup fresh parsley leaves, chopped
  - 1/4 cup fresh cilantro leaves, chopped
  - 3 cloves garlic, minced
  - 2 tablespoons red wine vinegar
  - 1/4 cup extra-virgin olive oil
  - 1/2 teaspoon dried oregano
  - 1/4 teaspoon red pepper flakes (optional)
  - Salt and pepper to taste

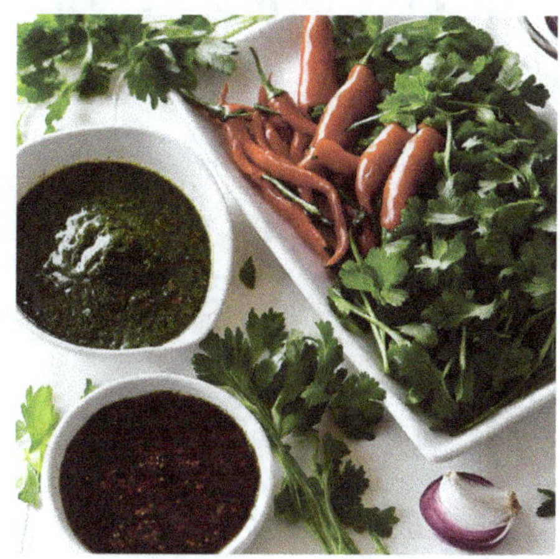

Procedure:
  1. In a small bowl, combine the chopped parsley leaves, chopped cilantro leaves, minced garlic, red wine vinegar, extra-virgin olive oil, dried oregano, and red pepper flakes (if using).
  2. Stir until well combined.
  3. Season with salt and pepper to taste, and stir again.
  4. Taste and adjust seasoning if needed.
  5. Use immediately as a sauce for grilled meats, roasted vegetables, or sandwiches, or store in an airtight container in the refrigerator for up to 1 week.

Nutritional values
(per tablespoon serving):
  - Calories: 40
  - Protein: 0g
  - Fat: 4g
  - Carbohydrates: 1g
  - Fiber: 0g

Shopping list:
  - Fresh parsley leaves
  - Fresh cilantro leaves
  - Garlic
  - Red wine vinegar
  - Extra-virgin olive oil
  - Dried oregano
  - Red pepper flakes (optional)
  - Salt
  - Pepper

98. Maple Dijon Dressing

- Preparation time: 5 minutes
- Cooking time: N/A
- Portions: Makes about 1/2 cup

Ingredients and quantity:
  - 3 tablespoons extra-virgin olive oil
  - 2 tablespoons apple cider vinegar
  - 1 tablespoon Dijon mustard
  - 1 tablespoon maple syrup
  - 1 clove garlic, minced
  - Salt and pepper to tast

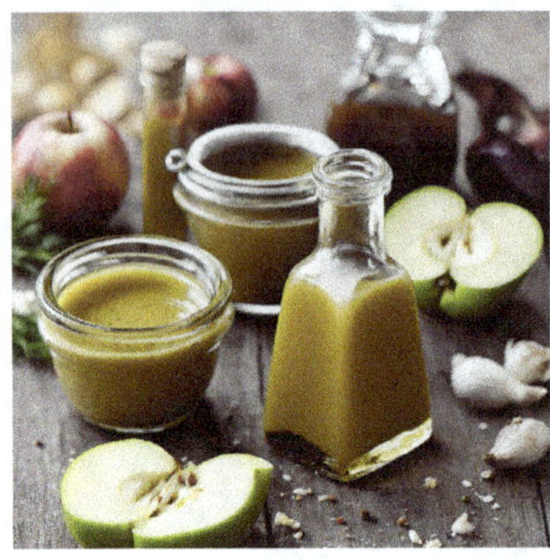

Procedure:
  1. In a small bowl, whisk together the extra-virgin olive oil, apple cider vinegar, Dijon mustard, maple syrup, and minced garlic until emulsified.
  2. Season with salt and pepper to taste, and whisk again until well combined.
  3. Taste and adjust seasoning if needed.
  4. Use immediately as a dressing for salads, roasted vegetables, or grain bowls, or store in an airtight container in the refrigerator for up to 1 week.

Nutritional values (per tablespoon serving):
  - Calories: 60
  - Protein: 0g
  - Fat: 7g
  - Carbohydrates: 2g
  - Fiber: 0g

Shopping list:

  - Extra-virgin olive oil
  - Apple cider vinegar
  - Dijon mustard
  - Maple syrup
  - Garlic
  - Salt
  - Pepper

99. Sriracha Mayo

- Preparation time: 5 minutes
- Cooking time: N/A
- Portions: Makes about 1/2 cup

Ingredients and quantity:
  - 1/2 cup vegan mayonnaise
  - 1 tablespoon sriracha sauce
    (adjust to taste)
  - 1 teaspoon lime juice
  - Salt to taste

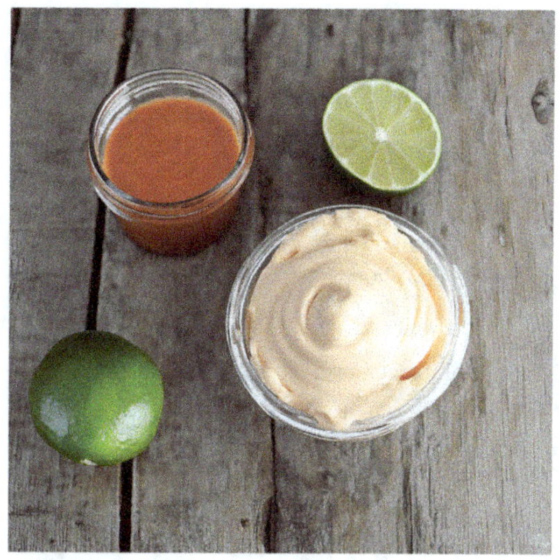

Procedure:
  1. In a small bowl, combine the vegan
     mayonnaise, sriracha sauce, and lime juice.
  2. Stir until well mixed.
  3. Season with salt to taste, and stir again.
  4. Taste and adjust the amount of sriracha sauce
     according to your preference for spiciness.
  5. Use immediately as a dipping sauce for fries, a spread for sandwiches, or a topping
     for burgers, or store in an airtight container in the refrigerator for up to 1 week.

Nutritional values (per tablespoon serving):
  - Calories: 50
  - Protein: 0g
  - Fat: 5g
  - Carbohydrates: 1g
  - Fiber: 0g

Shopping list:
  - Vegan mayonnaise
  - Sriracha sauce
  - Lime

100. Avocado Lime Crema

- Preparation time: 5 minutes
- Cooking time: N/A
- Portions: Makes about 1/2 cup

Ingredients and quantity:
  - 1 ripe avocado
  - 1/4 cup vegan sour cream or yogurt
  - 1 tablespoon lime juice
  - 1 tablespoon chopped cilantro (optional)

Procedure:
1. In a small bowl, mash the ripe avocado until smooth.
2. Add the vegan sour cream or yogurt and lime juice to the mashed avocado.
3. Stir until well combined.
4. If desired, mix in the chopped cilantro.
5. Season with salt and pepper to taste, and stir again.
6. Use immediately as a topping for tacos, salads, or grilled vegetables, or store in an airtight container in the refrigerator for up to 2 days.

- Salt and pepper to taste

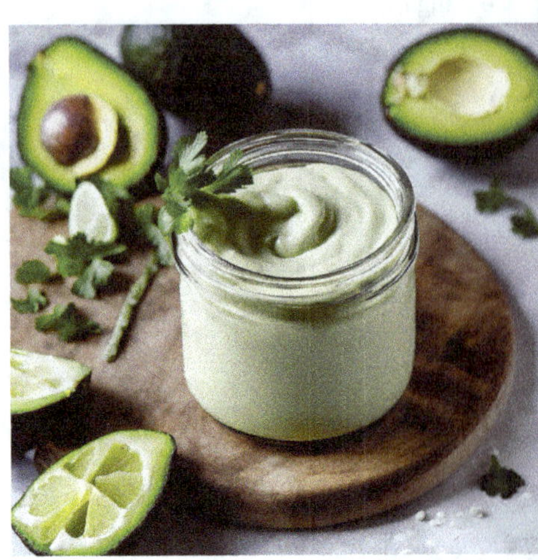

Nutritional values (per tablespoon serving):
  - Calories: 20
  - Protein: 0g
  - Fat: 2g
  - Carbohydrates: 1g
  - Fiber: 0g

Shopping list:
  - Ripe avocado
  - Vegan sour cream or yogurt
  - Lime
  - Cilantro (optional)
  - Salt
  - Pepper

As we reach the end of this culinary journey, it's clear that the marriage of health and flavor in plant-based cuisine is not only possible but also deeply satisfying. Through the exploration of vibrant ingredients, creative combinations, and nourishing recipes, we've uncovered the joy of cooking and eating in a way that nourishes both body and soul.

From hearty soups to refreshing salads, from wholesome grains to indulgent desserts, each dish has offered a glimpse into the endless possibilities of plant-based cooking. Along the way, we've discovered the beauty of seasonal produce, the richness of spices and herbs, and the art of mindful preparation.

But our journey doesn't end here. It continues as we bring these newfound skills and recipes into our daily lives, sharing them with loved ones and spreading the joy of healthy, delicious eating.

Whether you're a seasoned chef or a novice cook, I hope this book has inspired you to embrace the abundance of nature's bounty and explore the boundless flavors of plant-based cuisine.

As we bid farewell, let's remember that the kitchen is not just a place to prepare food, but a space for creativity, connection, and celebration.

So let's continue to savor the beauty of plant-based cooking, one delicious bite at a time.

Bon appétit, and may your journey to health and happiness be as rich and fulfilling as the flavors on your plate.

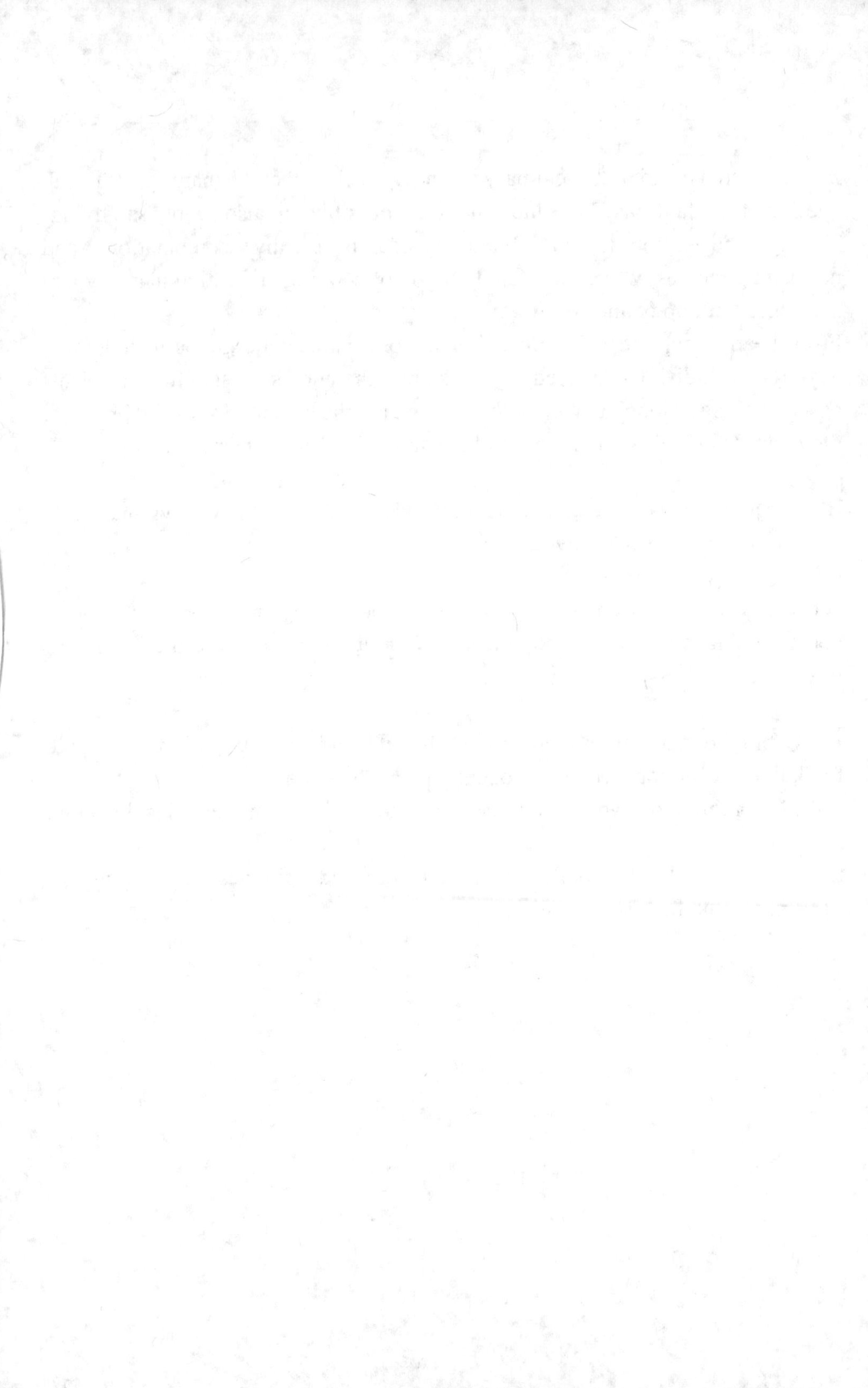